I0427046

SIMPLE STEPS
TO BOOST
HEALTH & ENERGY

On Your Way to A
Healthier You!

A COOKBOOK WITH

SIMPLE STEPS TO BOOST HEALTH & ENERGY!

EVERYDAY RECIPES, HEALTHIER INGREDIENTS!

By
Debra Schilling

For questions contact:
All He Says I Am
11127 Peach Ridge Ave.
Sparta, Mi. 49345

ISBN-13:978-1493552603
ISBN-10:1493552600

Cover design by *Debra K. Schilling*
Cover Photos by *Sonie Curtis*

*"I will Praise You, for I am fearfully and wonderfully made;
Marvelous are Your works, and that my soul knows very well."*
Psalm 139:14 NKJV

Table of Contents

Introduction   6

Health Notes   9

Everyday Health Habits   13

Foods to Avoid   14

Sweet Substitutes for Sugar   15

Food Facts   16

Breakfast, Muffins, Breads   17

Side Dishes   33

Main Dishes   53

Desserts   75

Snacks   93

Dips & spreads   103

Smoothies   113

Seasonings – Herbs & Spices   121

Glossary   127

Introduction

I love nutrition! It extends my life, gives me energy, makes my skin glow, makes me look younger (ok, maybe this is really why I like it), I feel better, therefore I'm happier, and I like happy. I sleep better, my mind is clearer, life is just... *better.*

I've always considered myself a healthy person, watching my fat intake, eating a fruit and vegetable a day. I exercised every day in one form or another. And I only had a dessert once a day.

Then in 2009 I started to have heart palpitations. They were so hard one night they woke me up. My doctor put me on blood pressure medication and one to lower my cholesterol. I never liked taking pills, not even vitamins so this was not fun. We lived at 9000 feet up in the Sacramento Mountains of New Mexico at the time. I told myself the health problems were a result of the high altitude. My body will get used to it... it never did. We lived there for five years.

So, I started studying healthy living via the internet, books, videos, etc. It didn't take long to see that the healthy living I thought I was doing was not all that healthy. Sugar, flour and processed foods were not on any healthy food list I found while doing researching. I had to make a change. I wanted to live a long life to see my children's children. And, I wanted my family to live long, healthy lives as well.

I stopped eating anything with refined sugar or flour in it and all processed food. Every morning I made myself a smoothie with spinach, kale, frozen blue berries, frozen strawberries, flax seed, apple and banana.

For lunch I would make a large salad with spinach, lettuce, nuts, sunflower seeds, dried cranberries, any fruit I had that wasn't frozen, tomato and cucumber. Sometimes I would slice an avocado (which was .50 cents each where we lived, sometimes 3 for $1) and use that for a dressing.

For dinner I ate fish or chicken, stir fried shredded carrots, Chinese lettuce (it's firm and sautes well), and/or shredded zucchini and yellow squash. The frying pan would be mounded with those veggies. And in all my food I would add a lot of spices and herbs.

Our finances were tight at that time and I was concerned about spending the extra money for all whole foods. But after about three weeks of buying food for me and food for my family, I noticed that our grocery bill had not gone up at all. How can this be? Everyone knows eating healthy cost more. So I added up how much I spent on food for me, figured out how much each meal would cost, added that up for each day and arrived at this figure, $5.80. I could hardly believe it! I checked my figures again, $5.80 a day. Costing too much to eat well was an old wives tale. It cost less to eat what I ate per day than what my *family* ate per day.

After three months or so I extended my eating habits to making bread, desserts and snacks that add to the per day cost. But it is far from the "it's so expensive to eat healthy" wives tale.

And, an unexpected plus to changing my eating habits was the weight I lost. I dropped thirty pounds in three months. My mind was so focused on being healthy and living a long life that I did not realize I was losing weight. The weather was turning cool and one morning I put on a pair of jeans, they were too big. What a surprise!

The more I study health, the more I'm amazed at how wonderfully we are made. I am convinced that our bodies were not created to consume unnatural substances. I heard once that healthy shopping is in the produce area of the grocery store and along the meat and dairy wall. The interior isles are the ones to avoid, save a few items.

There are so many "Simple Steps to Boost Health and Energy" that we can take, and every one will be worthwhile. This Cookbook takes everyday recipes and replaces ingredients with healthier ones. Start now, start small, start big, start completely... just start! *You can do it! I have faith in you!*

Health Notes

Our immune system thrives when we provide a nutritious, whole foods diet, plenty of high quality sleep, fresh clean filtered water, exercise, appropriate supplements and some form of stress management (walks on the beach, gardening, playing with your kids, reading, anything that brings rest and peace). Here is a list of Helps *for you. Most of these we do every day but with some simple changes you can improve your quality of living:*

- Adequate sleep is a lifestyle that is linked to good immunity.
- Keeping a positive attitude can affect our health for the better. A negative attitude can affect our health for the worst.
- Regular exercise, like a brisk 30-minute walk, is a good way to reduce stress and improve your overall health. It helps get more oxygen in your body and should be done every day.
- According to a study published in the American Journal of Preventive Medicine if you gargle (don't swallow) with plain water three times a day throughout cold and flu season you'll cut your risk of catching a cold by almost 40%.
- Treat dry, cracked lips with a layer of raw organic honey. The antibacterial properties of the honey help with healing. I have a dry spot on the side of my nose, right where my glasses rest. Sometimes it gets irritated so I put honey on it overnight. In the morning it's healed.

- If you're craving sweets try 1 tsp. of baking soda in 8 ounces of warm water. Rinse your mouth with the solution, but do not swallow. Your cravings will disappear for hours.
- Bad breath is often due to excessive dryness in your mouth. Make certain you're drinking lots of water not only to moisten the tissue inside your mouth but also to remove any small bits of food that may be lodged between your teeth.
- Another remedy for bad breath is eating a little plain yogurt. Be sure it does not contain sugar. The live bacteria in yogurt counteract the bacteria responsible for bad breath.
- Keep a bunch of ordinary or Italian parsley on hand. Chewing parsley after eating can naturally freshen your breath and serve as a mini-toothbrush.
- If you're troubled by indigestion, try combining 1 tsp. of lemon juice, 1 tsp. of ginger juice, and 2 tsp. of raw organic honey. Mix well, and drink it *after* a meal.
- Your digestive system breaks down food and delivers nutrients to cells throughout your body. Carbohydrates (from garden food, not noodles or breads), omega 3 fats (fish, oils, avocados, etc.) and proteins are key nutrients we obtain from food, along with fiber, water, vitamins, and minerals. By "food," I mean unprocessed, unrefined food as close to its natural state as possible. Processing and refining remove important substances, like fiber, vitamins, and minerals, and add ingredients that are not good for your body.
- Sugars, candy, donuts, cakes, chips, etc. have **no** nutrients and are sent to your cells to be stored. Your digestive system does not know what to do with them. Thus, weight is gained. Sugar also requires calcium for digestion therefore depleting necessary calcium for your bones.

- 1 cup of cooked kale contains 206 mg. of calcium. According to research at Creighton University in Omaha, Nebraska and Purdue University the absorbable calcium levels in kale equal or exceed the absorption levels of milk.
- Many foods and beverages (even raw vegetables) are packaged in plastic containing **bisphenol A (BPA)**, a hormone-disrupting chemical. Glass is preferable.
- If your store does not offer paper produce bags, try these options: paper lunch bags make good produce bags. Reusable fabric bags are available most everywhere and work well for shopping and food storage. Wash the bags frequently to prevent cross-contamination with bacteria.
- Ziploc plastic bags and Saran Wrap are BPA-free, according to the manufacturer. SC Johnson Glad plastic storage containers are also BPA-free, according to the manufacturer.
- Many canned goods and beverages contain BPA (bisphenol A), which leaches from the can straight into your food.
- Avoid prepared, packaged food whenever you can, it's likely to contain unnecessary fat, salt, sugar and stabilizing chemicals.
- Use baking powder that is aluminum free.
- Do not use artificial sweeteners if at all possible. Honey, agave nectar, pure maple syrup, stevia and Xylitol are natural sweeteners. Xylitol is toxic to animals and should be used sparingly for yourself.
- Evaporated organic cane juice is still "sugar".
- Use unsweetened almond milk, flax milk as substitutes for cow's milk. Goat milk is also a great alternative to cow's milk and is less allergenic, naturally homogenized, much easier to digest and rarely causes lactose intolerance.
- Store all nuts and flours in the freezer (i.e. amaranth, millet, almond, coconut, etc.) if they aren't to be used immediately.

- Do not use shortening or lard. Coconut oil can be used instead of these products. It is great for frying as it can withstand temps up to 140^0 F without losing any nutritional value. It also does not burn your food.
- The best liquid oils are coconut and olive oil. Also sunflower oil and safflower oil. All of them can be used for baking or frying. Real butter is also a good fat and contains vitamins A, E and K_2. It is better for you than margarine.
- Avoid vegetable or canola oil.
- Use sea salt or kosher salt. The recipes in this book call for sea salt.
- Braggs Aminos is used in these recipes in place of soy sauce.

My Every Day Health Habits

• **Organic Apple Cider Vinegar** - ½ tsp. of organic Apple Cider Vinegar (I use Braggs) in 16 oz. of purified water every day, you can do once in the morning and once in the evening. Always take apple cider vinegar in water. It is like lemons which can strip your teeth of enamel if taken without water and in large doses.

•**Unrefined Coconut Oil** - Have 1 tbl. in oatmeal or any other food once a day. I will sometimes use 1 tbl. of coconut oil in hot purified water with honey and cinnamon.

•**Water** - Drink one ounce of water for every two pounds of weight. We lose water through skin evaporation, breathing, urine, and stool. These losses should be replaced.

• **Smoothie** – I use greens (spinach & kale), berries, banana, apple, walnuts. Add other fruit & flax seed if you like. Smoothies are a quick way to get a lot of nutrition in your body. Liquids can enter your system quicker than chewing your food.

• **Turmeric** – sprinkle on fish, meat or put in your smoothie. Turmeric is an anti-inflammatory and provides many health benefits including immune system, liver function, and joint support, flatulence, jaundice, menstrual difficulties, bloody urine, toothache and much more.

• **Honey & Cinnamon** – drink hot purified water with 1 tbl. honey and 1 tsp. cinnamon twice a day or just the cinnamon and honey mixed together. It satisfies a sweet craving.

Foods to Avoid

• Sugar, brown sugar, corn syrup, high fructose corn syrup, packaged sugar substitutes (the ones on restaurant tables). (Refined sugar has been depleted of its life forces, vitamins and minerals. What is left consists of pure, refined carbohydrates.)

• White flour, whole wheat flour, white rice (Modern commercial flour, especially white flour, has been stripped of the parts of the wheat kernel that slow its digestion; it's extremely easy for the body to turn white flour into blood sugar).

• Cereals – they all have some form of sugar

• Potato and corn chips

• Cookies, candies, cakes, pastries

• Pasta

 • Anything low fat, no fat, skim (they replace with sugar)

• All processed meat

• Most canned foods as they contain sugar, read labels.

Sweet Substitutes For Sugar

• Bananas

• Applesauce

• Honey

• Pure Maple Syrup

• Agave Nectar

• Xilatol - found in health food Store, is poison for animals, use sparingly for yourself.

• Raw Stevia - without additional ingredients, found in health food store.

• Turbonado Sugar – from partially refine sugar cane extract. Found in health food stores.

Food Facts

Artery-Cleansing Foods
Avocados, Olive Oil, Coconut Oil, Walnuts, Almonds, Salmon, Broccoli, Asparagus, Turmeric, Persimmons, Cinnamon, Pure Honey, Cranberries, Green Tea, Spinach

Bone Health Foods
No dairy except: Yogurt, Whole Cream, Sour Cream, Cottage Cheese and Butter. Eggs, Onion, Garlic, Tart Red Cherries

Brain Health Foods
Black Berries, Apples, Cinnamon, Spinach, Coconut oil, Olive Oil, Salmon, Curry, Concord Grape Juice, Dark Green leafy Vegetables, Avocado, Sunflower Seeds

Arthritis, Anti Inflammatory
Salmon, Walnuts, Pumpkin Seeds, Flax Seed, Extra Virgin Olive Oil, Coconut Oil, Sweet Peppers, Onions and Leeks, Tart Cherries

Breakfast, Muffins, Breads

Debra's Pancakes Mix	18
Almond Meal Pancakes	19
Healthy Pancake Mix	19
Banana Pancakes	20
Pancake Apple Rings	20
Pumpkins Waffles	21
Sweet Pepper Frittata	22
Turkey Breakfast Frittata	23
Egg Custard Pudding	23
Eggs in Pepper Rings	24
Avocado Focaccia & Egg Breakfast	24
Breakfast Cookies	25
Almond Butter Banana Muffins	26
Baked Oatmeal	27
Pumpkin Bread	28
Chickpea Flat Bread	29
Flax seed Focaccia Bread	30

Debra's Pancake Mix

½ c. oats, whole   1 tbl. sunflower seeds; roasted

Directions:
Place oats and sunflower seeds in a blender or grinder (I use a
$15 grinder I bought at Walmart) with sunflower seeds on top and
grind. I use the fine setting on my grinder. This recipe will make 3
– 4 small pancakes. I pour honey on top my pancakes instead of
syrup. I also make up several batches of enough mix to store in an
airtight container in my cupboard. It's ready to use! Several
recipes in this book call for this "flour".

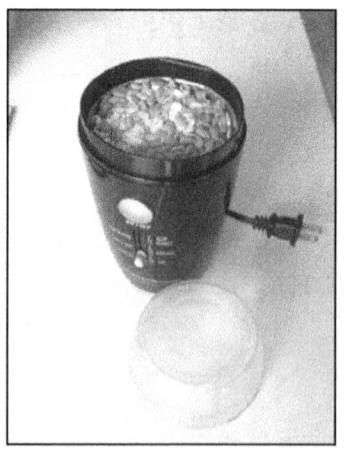

My Grinder from Walmart

Almond Meal Pancakes

3 lg. eggs ⅛ tsp. vanilla extract
1 c. almond meal (flour) ⅛ tsp. ground cinnamon
½ tbl. butter or olive, coconut, sunflower oil

Directions:
In a medium bowl mix eggs with a fork until well blended. Add the almond meal mixing as you add. Add vanilla and cinnamon, mix well. Spoon the batter into a buttered or oiled skillet (olive oil, coconut oil, sunflower oil). Cook over medium to medium-low heat until both sides are golden brown. Drizzle with raw honey. Add fruit to your liking or spread with almond butter. I suggest small pancakes; they tend to stick together if they are large.

Healthy Pancake Mix

½ c. old fashioned oatmeal 1 tsp. vanilla
1½ tbl. sunflower seeds ⅛tsp. baking soda
⅓c. water ½ tbl. olive oil
1 egg

Directions:
Grind oatmeal & sunflower seeds in coffee grinder. Place in a small bowl. Add the water and mix with a fork to avoid lumps. Add the egg, vanilla and baking soda one at a time, mix well. Spoon mixture into a medium sized fry pan with oil on medium heat. When the edges appear dry and bubbles form on top, flip. Makes 5 medium size pancakes. Top with fruit or honey.

Banana Pancakes

3 bananas   fruit of choice for topping

Directions:
Mash bananas until no lumps are left. Spoon onto an oiled fry pan, flip when the top appears dry, that's it! Really! They're great! Top with your favorite fruit.

Pancake Apple Rings

(Pan-fried)

3 green or red apples   1 tbl. olive oil
1 c. Healthy Pancake Mix   1 tbl. stevia

Directions:
Core apples and slice horizontally to make rings, 1/4 inch thick. Mix stevia with Healthy Pancake Mix. Dip apples in mix and fry in pan with olive oil until golden, flip till golden. Good with honey over the top. They are fun to make and are a pretty presentation.

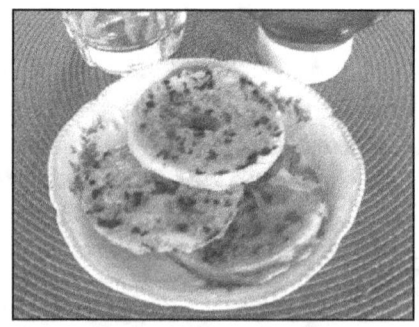

Apple Rings

Pumpkin Waffles

2 c. amaranth flour
2 c. rolled oats
1 30 oz. can pumpkin
¼ c. sunflower oil
2 tsp. cinnamon

1 tsp. nutmeg & sea salt
1 ½ tsp. baking powder
1 c. greek yogurt
2 tsp. vanilla
3 eggs

Directions:
Preheat a waffle maker. Place rolled oats in blender for 3 or 4 pulses to break them down, mix with almond meal, yogurt & water with a fork then cover and let sit overnight in fridge (optional). In the morning add the remaining ingredients and mix just until blended, not over mixing. Batter is dense and baking time usually is longer than waffle timer indicates. Top with fruit or yogurt.

Sweet Pepper Frittata

Preheat oven to 350°

1 sm. onion
¾ c. green pepper
¾ c. red pepper
½ c. sun dried tomatoes
2 tbl. butter
5 eggs, lightly beaten

½ c. sun dried tomatoes
1 ½ c. feta cheese
1 tsp. Braggs soy sauce
¼ tsp. black pepper
½ tsp. sea salt

Directions:
Chop onion, green & red pepper & dried tomatoes. Sauté onion & peppers in butter for 5-7 min, mix the remaining ingredients in a bowl until eggs are well mixed. Add sautéed veggies into the bowl mixture, pour into ungreased pie dish and bake for 25-30 minutes or until a knife inserted comes out clean. A yummy breakfast on cool mornings.

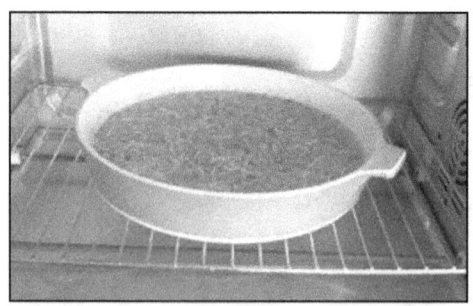

Sweet Pepper Frittata

Turkey Breakfast Frittata

½ med. onion, minced
4 med. cloves garlic, chopped
¼ lb. ground lamb or turkey
salt & pepper to taste

1 + 2 tbl. chicken broth
3 c. kale, chopped
5 eggs

Directions:
Preheat broiler on low. Heat 1 tbl. broth in a oven safe skillet, sauté onion over med. heat for about 3 min. stirring often. Add garlic, ground meat & cook for another 3 min. on med. breaking up clumps. Add kale & 2 tbl. of broth. Reduce heat to low, continue cooking covered for 5 min. Beat eggs in separate bowl, season with salt & pepper, pour on top of mixture. Cook on low for 2 min. Place skillet under broiler on High (my broiler has high and low) in middle of oven about 7 inches from heat source. As soon as eggs are firm, it's done, about 2-3 minutes. Nice meal for company brunch.

Egg Custard Pudding

Preheat oven to 400°

6 eggs
3 c. flax or almond milk
½ c. honey

1 tsp. vanilla extract
¼ tsp. sea salt
ground nutmeg

Directions:
Crack eggs and whip together in a shallow baking dish. Whisk in milk and honey. Add vanilla and salt, mix well. Bake in the same dish for 45 to 50 minutes or until bubbly on top and knife comes out clean. Serve warm or cold in custard cups with nutmeg sprinkled on top! It's almost like a dessert!

Eggs in Pepper Rings

1 green, red or yellow bell pepper
1 tbl. olive, sunflower or coconut oil

3 eggs
salt & pepper

Directions:
Slice pepper horizontally to make rings. Cut away seeds and place in fry pan on low to medium heat with oil for 30 seconds or so, flip for 15 seconds. Break an egg into each ring, sprinkle with salt & pepper to taste and turn to low heat. Cook slowly until desired doneness. You get a veggie along with your egg. You could sprinkle with a little cilantro or parsley. It makes a pretty presentation!

Avocado Focaccia & Egg Breakfast

1 avocado
1 tbl. onion, chopped
1 tbl. tomato, chopped
1 tsp. garlic powder

salt & pepper to taste
½ tbl. lime juice
2 lg. eggs
1 piece Focaccia Flax Bread

Directions:
Cut avocado in half, turning as you slice through, to the seed. Scoop out the meat with a spoon. Mix the avocado meat with the chopped onion, tomato, garlic powder, salt & pepper and lime juice together in a small bowl (like you're making guacamole), and set aside. Fry eggs over easy or poached. Meanwhile, place Flax seed Focaccia Bread slice (pg.30) on a plate and spread with the avocado mix. Place eggs on top of avocado mix and ENJOY!!! One of my favorites!

Breakfast Cookies

Preheat oven to 350º

1 ½ c. regular rolled oats
¼ c. almond meal
½ c. mixed nuts, chopped
1 c. coconut flakes
½ tsp. allspice
½ tsp. salt

1 tsp. cinnamon
1 c. dried fruit of choice
¼ c. olive oil
3 c. ripe bananas, mashed
1 tsp. vanilla extract

Directions:
Line a baking sheet with parchment paper. In a large bowl combine rolled oats, almond meal, mixed nuts and coconut flakes. Stir in allspice, salt & cinnamon, add dried fruit, stir until evenly mixed. In bowl mix oil, mashed bananas & vanilla, pour this mixture over dry ingredients, stir well. Using a spoon, place batter onto a cookie sheet, not touching cookies together. Bake for 20 minutes or until edges are golden brown. A nice treat when the kids come home from school. Their "meaty", satisfying and my husband's favorite!

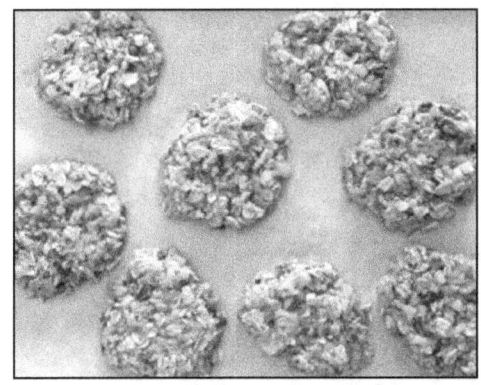

Breakfast Cookie

Almond Butter Banana Muffins

Preheat oven to 350º

3 ripe bananas, mashed
¼ c. almond butter
⅓ c. Stevia
1 egg white
1 tsp. vanilla
1 ½ c. amaranth flour

1 tsp. baking powder
½ tsp. baking soda
½ tsp. salt
½ c. dark unsweetened
   choco. chips
½ c. chopped pecans

Directions:
Mix bananas, almond butter, stevia, egg white & vanilla until creamy. Stir in flour, baking powder, soda & salt. Add choco chips and pecans. Place in paper lined muffin cups, bake for 20 minutes or until knife comes out clean.

Baked Oatmeal

Preheat oven 375°

1 lb. old-fashioned oats
1 c. walnuts
2 tbl. greek yogurt
dash sea salt
6 eggs
2 c. almond or flax milk

¼ c. honey
½ c. dried cranberries
½ c. dried apricots,
2 tbl. cinnamon
¼ c. coconut oil
water

Directions:
Mix oats and walnuts in a bowl, add enough filtered water to cover, add greek yogurt & salt, soak overnight in fridge. In the morning drain oats in colander, return to bowl. In a separate bowl beat eggs, milk, honey until frothy, pour over the oats & nuts stir well. Fold in fruit, cinnamon and coconut oil, pour into greased 13 x 9 baking pan smoothing it out. Bake 40 to 45 min., until the top is golden brown and inserted knife comes out clean. Cool for 5 minutes then cut into squares and enjoy! Add whipped whole cream and fruit on top!

Pumpkin Bread

Preheat oven to 375º

¾ c. amaranth flour
½ tsp. of baking powder, soda, salt
¾ tsp. cinnamon
½ tsp. ground cloves

3 lg. eggs
1 c. honey
1 c. pumpkin puree
⅔ c. regular oats

Directions:
Oil a loaf pan or 3 mini loaf pans or a muffin tin. Combine amaranth flour, baking powder, soda, salt, cinnamon and cloves in a small bowl. Beat eggs and honey in a large bowl until combined, stir in pumpkin, then flour mixture, then oats. Pour into loaf pan(s) and bake 25 to 30 minutes in a single loaf pan, 20 to 25 in mini loaves and 10 to 15 in muffin tin. Pumpkin, my favorite fall squash!

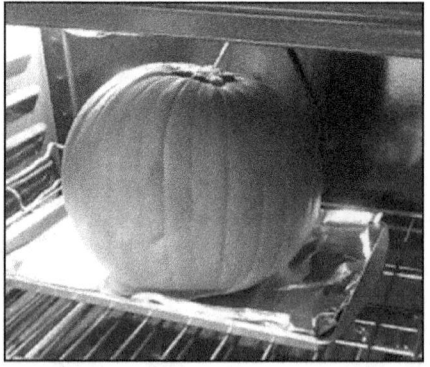

Cooking Pumpkin – 200° for 2 hr's or so.
The pumpkin will slump when done.
Cut top off, scoop out seeds, then meat. *So easy*!

Chickpea Flat Bread

Preheat oven to 350°

2 ½ c. garbanzo bean flour

3 ½ c. fresh cold water

1 tsp. salt & pepper to taste

¼ c. olive oil or sunflower oil

Directions:

A few hours before dinner put flour in a bowl & slowly add water, whisk to avoid lumps. Add salt & pepper as desired. Let mixture set for 2 or 3 hours. When it's time to cook, skim off the froth that forms with a slotted spoon. Pour olive oil on a large rimmed cookie sheet; pour the batter on top of the oil. The oil will move to the sides. Place in the pre-heated oven for 30 minutes, or until golden. Let it cool before cutting & serve. Sometimes I will add Italian seasoning & garlic powder to the mix. For another variation add 2 tbl. of honey for a sweet bread flavor.

Flax Seed Focaccia Bread

Preheat oven to 350°

2 c. flax seed meal
½ tsp. baking soda
½ tsp. salt
4 tbl. honey

5 lg. eggs, beaten
½ c. water
⅓ c. coconut or olive oil

Directions:
Mix all the dry ingredients with a whisk. In a separate bowl mix all the wet ingredients well with a whisk. Slowly add dry ingredients to the wet ingredients, mixing as you are adding. Let the mixture set for 3 to 5 min. Place dough on an oiled rimmed cookie sheet or a round rimmed pizza pan and spread out with a spoon. Bake for 20 minutes, until the bread springs back when touched. This is so good; you won't know its flax seed meal. It's one of my favorites! I cut the bread into squares and freeze two pieces in a zip lock bag. Try spreading hummus on top or toasting a piece with butter on top!!!!

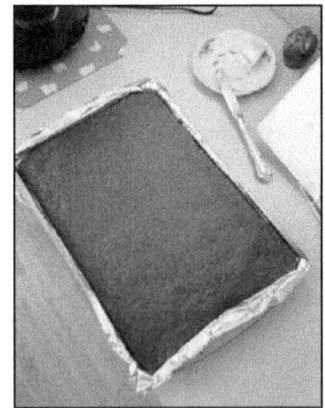

Flax Seed Focaccia Bread

Notes

_____

_____

_____

_____

_____

_____

_____

_____

_____

_____

_____

_____

_____

_____

_____

_____

_____

_____

_____

_____

_____

_____

_____

Notes

_____

_____

_____

_____

_____

_____

_____

_____

_____

_____

_____

_____

_____

_____

_____

_____

_____

_____

_____

_____

_____

_____

_____

Sides

Raw Applesauce, Quick	34
Apple Sauce, Crock Pot	34
Autumn Coleslaw	35
Autumn Chopped Salad	35
Italian Broccoli	36
Cheesy Cauliflower Pancakes	36
Mashed Cauliflower	37
Roasted Curried Cauliflower	37
Crab Salad	38
Cucumber Rollups	39
Deviled Eggs	39
Baked Parmesan Green Beans	40
Orange Cranberry Squash	41
Turkey Waldorf Salad	42
Italian Tomatoes (Pizza Tomatoes)	42
Spaghetti Squash in White Sauce	43
Pumpkin Apple Sauce	44
Sweet Potato Rounds	44
Spiced Potato Rounds	45
Garlic Parmesan Potatoes	45
Vegetable Medley	46
Zucchini Boats	47
Zucchini Sticks, Baked	48
Zucchini Potato Pancakes	48
"Fried" Zucchini Sticks	49
Zucchini Noodles	50

Raw Applesauce, Quick

1 c. water   ⅓ c. lemon juice
2 tsp. nutmeg   2 tsp. cinnamon
4 large Jonathan or Fuji apples cored/quartered
⅓ c. or more, to taste, pure maple syrup

Directions:
Pulse all ingredients in a blender, blend until it's a chunky sauce.
Or, blend until puréed for saucy sauce. Eat. Oh, I love quick and
good! Triple the recipe and put some in your freezer!

Apple Sauce, Crock Pot

15 small apples, Honey Crisp is wonderful
cinnamon

Directions:
Core and chop apples in small pieces. I leave the skins on. (If you
don't like the skins, core and peel, slice in quarters) Place in crock
pot on high for about 4 hours. Sprinkle cinnamon on top and stir.
Place in freezer zip lock bags. So easy and so good!

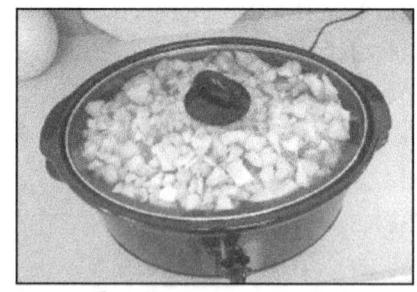

Applesauce ready to cook!

Autumn Coleslaw

¼ c. greek yogurt
¼ c. sour cream
1 tbl. apple cider vinegar
3 tsp. honey
¼ tsp. celery seed

⅛ tsp. salt
3 c. cabbage, shredded
1 c. carrot, shredded
½ c. radishes, sliced
¾ c. onion, chopped

Directions:
Combine yogurt, sour cream, vinegar, honey, celery seed & salt.
Toss with cabbage, carrot, radishes & onion.
For another version: _omit_ vinegar, celery seed, & radishes. _Add_ 1
tbl. Dijon mustard, 1 c. chopped apple, red or green (both is pretty)
and 1 c. shredded fresh spinach. The taste of fall!

Autumn Chopped Salad

6 to 7 c. romaine, chopped
2 med. pears, chopped
1 c. dried cranberries
1 c. pecans, chopped
balsamic vinaigrette & poppy seed dressing

3 c. cabbage, shredded
8 slices bacon crisp
4 to 5 slices feta cheese

Directions:
On a large platter or bowl combine all ingredients and drizzle with
poppy seed dressing and some balsamic vinaigrette. Oh, my
goodness, this is good! It has a cozy taste!

Italian Broccoli

Preheat oven to 425°

2 lg. bunches of broccoli cut into florets
5 tbl. olive oil   1 ½ tsp. kosher or sea salt
½ tsp. ground pepper   4 garlic cloves, sliced
⅓ c. promising cheese   lemon

Directions:
Rinse broccoli & drain thoroughly, toss in bowl with 3 ½ tbl. oil, salt, pepper & garlic. Place on cookie sheet and roast until crisp-tender, about 20-25 min. shaking pan around a few times to turn florets. Remove and zest lemon over florets, then squeeze lemon liquid over florets. Toss with 1 ½ tbl. of oil and add parmesan cheese. *Delicious!*

Cheesy Cauliflower Pancakes

1 head cauliflower   ½ c. Panco bread crumbs
2 lg. eggs   ½ tsp. cayenne pepper
½ c. italian blend cheese   pinch of salt, oil

Directions:
Cut cauliflower into florets & cook in boiling water until tender, about 10 min. Drain & mash cauliflower with a fork while still warm. Add beaten eggs, cheese, bread crumbs, cayenne & salt to taste. Coat a griddle or skillet with olive oil over medium-high heat. Form cauliflower mixture into 3" patties and cook until golden brown & firm to flip, about 3 minutes per side. Makes 8 pancakes. Oh, oh… mouth watering!

Mashed Cauliflower

1 bag frozen cauliflower or 1 small head
¼ c. parmesan cheese   ¼ tsp. garlic powder
½ bar cream cheese   salt & pepper to taste

Directions:
Cook cauliflower until soft. If you use a head of cauliflower, take off leaves and place in large pot with 2 inches of water, cover and cook till soft, about 20 minutes adding more water if needed. I steam cauliflower in a rice/veggie steamer. Place soft cauliflower in a bowl and add remaining ingredients, puree with immersion blender or potato masher. And enjoy, so good!

Roasted Curried Cauliflower

Preheat oven to 500°

1 head cauliflower   curry powder
olive oil   kosher or sea salt

Directions:
Break cauliflower into medium-small florets & place into large bowl or baking pan. Size pieces evenly or they will cook unevenly. Drizzle cauliflower pieces well with olive oil and season with salt and curry powder. Place in single layer on cookie sheet. Cover pan with foil and roast until florets are soft & translucent looking, about 10-15 minutes Remove foil and toss florets with tongs, roast 30-35 minutes more until crisp, tossing every 8-10 minutes. A cool weather delight!

Crab Salad

2 pkg. imitation crab
2 c. sour cream
2 tbl. olive oil
½ tsp. dijon mustard

2 celery stalks, chopped
½ onion, chopped
salt & pepper

Directions:
Break crab into smaller pieces in a medium size bowl. In a small bowl mix sour cream, olive oil and Dijon mustard. Add celery and onion, salt & pepper. Mix well and chill. It's ready to serve and so good!

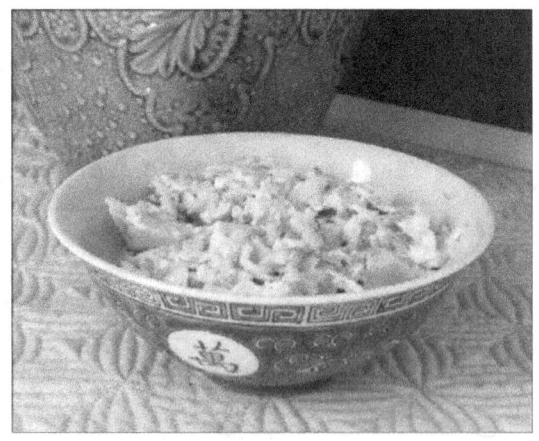

Crab Salad

Cucumber Rollups

1 cucumber
hummus
salt & pepper
sliced ham or turkey

shredded white cheese
curry powder or turmeric
cilantro (optional)

Directions:
Slice cucumber very thin lengthwise. Spread hummus on cucumber slices, sprinkle with salt and pepper. Place your meat choice on top and sprinkle on cheese, curry or turmeric and cilantro. Roll up and secure with a tooth pick. So good and refreshing! You can leave out the meat if you prefer.

Deviled Eggs

6 eggs
¼ c. sour cream
1 tsp. mustard
¼ tsp. salt & pepper

¼ tsp. apple cider vinegar
½ tsp. olive oil
Paprika

Directions:
Boil eggs for 12 minutes. When done place pan under cold running water for 3 minutes or so, until pan and eggs are cool. In a small bowl mix sour cream, mustard, salt & pepper, apple cider vinegar and oil together. Shell eggs, cut in half lengthwise and remove yoke with a spoon. Add sour cream mixture. Spoon mixture into egg halves and sprinkle with paprika. Ta da!

Baked Parmesan Green Beans

Preheat oven to 400º

8 oz. or 1 pkg. frozen green beans
1 tbl. olive oil
salt & pepper

parmesan cheese
3 slices bacon

Directions:
Cook bacon till crisp, break into pieces. Place green beans with ends trimmed off in a medium bowl, sprinkle with oil, salt & pepper to taste. Sprinkle with crumbled bacon. Mix well. Lay green beans on a cookie sheet and sprinkle a healthy amount of cheese on top, I like a lot. Bake for 15 to 20 minutes. Beans should be crisp on the outside and tender on the inside. This is a nice side dish for a holiday meal. Enjoy!

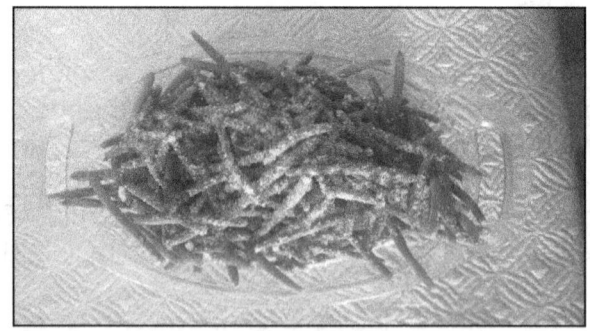

Baked Parmesan Green Beans

Orange Cranberry Squash

Preheat oven to 400°

1 acorn squash, any size

⅓ c. Xylitol

½ tsp. cinnamon

5 c. frozen or fresh cranberries

4 oranges or clementine's

1 tsp. butter

½ c. water

Directions:

Cut squash in half lengthwise and scoop out seeds, prick squash with a fork, place skin side down on a baking pan that has been lined with tin foil. In a bowl mix the Xylitol and cinnamon together, add cranberries and toss. Spoon the mixture into the squash and arrange orange sections on top, add a small amount of butter. Pour water into the pan, cover squash with tin foil and bake for about an hour until squash is tender. You can pour juices that are left in the pan over the squash and serve, cause its soooo good!

Turkey Waldorf Salad

1 green apple
1 red delicious apple
½ c. pineapple juice, unsweetened
½ lb. cooked turkey, diced
¾ c. celery, diced

¼ c. sour cream
¾ c. greek yogurt, plain
2 tbl. honey or to taste
3 tbl. chopped walnuts

Directions:
Core and chop the apples, soak in pineapple juice for 2 min. drain & discard juice. Add to bowl turkey and celery. Whisk together sour cream, yogurt & honey, pour over turkey, apples, celery & toss. Garnish with walnuts. This is a refreshing summer taste!

Italian Tomatoes (or Pizza Tomatoes)

2 firm tomatoes
1 c. parmesan cheese
1 tbl. italian seasoning

1 tbl. garlic
salt & pepper to taste

Directions:
Slice tomatoes less than ¼ inch thick and place on tin foil lined cookie sheet. Mix parmesan cheese, Italian seasoning, garlic, salt & pepper together and sprinkle on top of tomatoes and bake till topping is lightly browned, about 10 minutes. My family loves these!

Spaghetti Squash in White Sauce

Preheat oven to 375º

1 lg. spaghetti squash
4 slices bacon, chopped
2 tsp. minced garlic
¼ c. chicken broth

2 egg yolks + 1 egg
1 c. parmesan cheese
2 tsp. salt
1 ¼ tsp. pepper

Directions:
Prick the squash all over with a fork. Roast on a foil lined pan 1 1/2 hours, till sides of squash start to sag. Let cool a bit. Slice in half lengthwise, scoop out seeds then scoop out squash with a fork and place in a large bowl. Fry the chopped bacon in a pan until crispy. Add the garlic and sauté for 1 minute. Add the broth and cook until the liquid has completely evaporated. In a medium bowl, whisk the eggs together with the cheese. Season with the salt & pepper. Combine the eggs with the bacon mixture, stir to just warm the eggs in the pan (do not let the eggs cook through). Add the spaghetti squash and toss to thoroughly combine and until squash is heated through. Adjust seasoning if necessary and serve. A nice Sunday family side dish!

Pumpkin Apple Sauce

Preheat oven to 350º

2 ½ lbs. apples, cored & chopped
2 tsp. ground cinnamon
juice of 1 lemon

¾ c. water
½ c. pumpkin puree
1 tsp. vanilla

Directions:
In heavy bottomed pot heat apples, cinnamon, lemon juice and water. The liquid will not cover the apples, bring to a boil then lower heat and simmer for 45 minutes to an hour stirring occasionally until apples are soft. Once soft, remove from heat. For chunky sauce add pumpkin puree and vanilla, smash apples with a potato masher to desired chunkiness. For smooth sauce, blend apples in a blender, pumpkin puree and vanilla until… smooth. Freeze or serve… or eat right now!

Sweet Potato Rounds

Preheat oven to 350º

2 sweet potatoes, sliced ¼ inch thick

1 tbl. olive oil

Directions:
Brush sliced potatoes on both sides with olive oil and place on parchment lined cookie sheet. Bake for 20 minutes. Turn heat to 400º and bake for 15 to 20 minutes more. You can sprinkle with honey and cinnamon if you like but it is SO great just the way they are.

Spiced Potato Rounds

Preheat oven to 450°

2 potatoes	garlic powder
1 tbl. olive oil	salt & pepper to taste
italian seasoning	1 tbl. parmesan cheese

Directions:
Slice potatoes very thin, less than ¼ inch. Toss with oil, Italian seasoning, garlic, salt & pepper in a zip lock bag to coat. Place on parchment lined cookie sheet and bake for 15 to 20 minutes. Sprinkle on cheese and bake for additional 5 minutes. A quick and fun dish!

Garlic Parmesan Potatoes

Crock Pot

3 lbs. yellow potatoes	2 tbl. parsley, chopped
½ tsp. baisl	2 tbl. olive oil
4 cloves of garlic	2 tbl. butter
½ tsp. oregano	¼ c. parmesan cheese

Directions:
Wash potatoes and microwave 5 at a time till not quite done, 5 min. or so. Meanwhile, in a large zip lock bag place the rest of the ingredients except the butter. Cut the potatoes in quarters, place in bag and shake around until all are coated. Place potatoes in crock pot, put cut up tbs of butter on top and cook on low for 4 hours.

Vegetable Medley

Preheat oven to 400°

1 tbl. olice oil
1 tsp. minced garlic
1 med. yellow onion, diced
1 med. zucchini
1 med. yellow squash

1 med. tomato
1 med. potato
1 tsp. dried thyme
salt & pepper to taste
1 c. shredded Italian cheese

Directions:
Sauté minced garlic and diced onion until softened. Meanwhile slice zucchini, squash, potato, tomato. Lightly oil a 9x9 pan, spread the onion garlic mixture on the bottom. Alternately stand the vegetable slices next to each other in the pan. Should make 4 rows. Sprinkle thyme, salt & pepper and cheese on top. Bake covered with foil for 30 minutes uncover and cook another 15 minutes or so until tender. Not only does it taste good, it makes a pretty presentation!

Zucchini Boats

Preheat oven to 350º

4 zucchini
2 roma tomatoes, chopped
1 tsp. italian seasoning
½ tsp. salt & pepper

½ tsp. garlic powder
½ c. white cheese
fresh parsley leaves

Directions:
Cut zucchini in half lengthwise and scoop out the seeds. Scoop out some of the zucchini meat leaving ¼ to ½ inch sides. Chop zucchini meat and place in a bowl. Lay boats on flat pan lined with aluminum foil. Mix the chopped tomatoes, italian seasoning, salt & pepper and garlic powder with extra zucchini meat. Place in boats. Sprinkle cheese and parsley on top. Bake for 15 to 20 minutes, until zucchini is soft but not mushy. Serve with a smile!

Zucchini Sticks, Baked

Preheat oven to 425º

1 lb. of zucchini
salt
½ c. cornmeal
¼ c. parmesan cheese
1 egg lightly beaten

Dipping Sauce:
½ c. greek yogurt
4 tbl. water
3 cloves garlic, mashed

Directions:
Cut zucchini in half, cut the halves into six sticks, season with salt. Mix cornmeal with parmesan cheese and place on a plate. Place beaten egg in a shallow bowl. Dip zucchini sticks in egg then coat with the cornmeal mixture. Place on a baking sheet, not touching each other. Bake until golden, about 25 minutes. Mix the rest of the ingredients for a dipping sauce; greek yogurt, water and garlic. Serve the sticks warm with the sauce. A good movie night munchie!

Zucchini Potato Pancakes

1 large potato
½ zucchini
⅛ c. parmesan cheese
⅛ c. monterey jack cheese

1 tsp. garlic powder
salt & pepper to taste
1 egg, beaten

Directions:
Grate potato and zucchini into hash brown consistency into a bowl, not using the zucchini seeds. Add cheeses and spices, mix well. Add beaten egg, mix well again. Form into patties and fry in olive oil a few minutes on each side, till golden. So yummy!

"Fried" Zucchini Sticks

Preheat oven to 425°

¼ c. olive oil, 3 tbl. olive oil
2 lg. egg whites
¾ c. Panko bread crumbs
3 tbl. parmesan cheese

¾ tsp. italian seasoning
¼ tsp. salt
2 med. zucchini

Directions:
Oil rimmed baking sheet. Put egg whites in shallow dish, beat lightly. In another shallow dish mix Panko, cheese, Italian seasoning and salt. Cut zucchini in half, cut the halves lengthwise into 16 1" wedges. Dip zucchini in egg whites, one at a time, letting excess drip off. Roll in crumbs, pressing them so they adhere. Arrange close together but not touching on prepared pan. Drizzle with remaining 3 tablespoons oil. Bake without turning, 25 to 30 minutes, until zucchini is crisp and golden. Serve with marinara sauce for dipping. Goes great with the "Italian Tomatoes"!

Zucchini Noodles

1 zucchini per person
1 tbl. of butter
shallots

garlic
your favorite seasonings

Directions:
Peel zucchini with a potato peeler (skin and all) When you get down to the seeds, stop and throw them away. Slice pieces lengthwise into strips making noodles. Sauté them in the butter with seasonings, garlic and shallots. They cook quickly. You're going to be amazed how good these are. Top with cheese and/or marinara sauce. A great replacement for pasta noodles. I like to use an italian seasoning mixture sometimes. They make a nice side dish with pork steak!

Notes

Notes

_____

_____

_____

_____

_____

_____

_____

_____

_____

_____

_____

_____

_____

_____

_____

_____

_____

_____

_____

_____

_____

_____

Main Dishes

Crusted Tilapia	54
Baked/Grilled Salmon	54
Grilled Salmon with Avocado Salsa	55
Baked Salmon	56
Cauliflower Crust Pizza	57
Zesty Chicken Kabobs	57
Honey Sauced Chicken	58
Loaded Chicken or Tuna Salad	59
Roasted Chicken Salad w/Almonds	59
Thai Chicken	60
Chicken Tacos, Crock Pot	60
Honey Chicken, Crock Pot	61
Coconut Chicken	61
Honey Lime Shrimp	62
Lemon Butter Shrimp	62
Quinoa Burgers	63
Zucchini Pizza	63
Taco Roll Ups	64
Ratatouille	65
Sweet Potato Cauliflower Soup	66
Tomato/Avocado Pizza	67
Asparagus Soup	68
Butternut Squash Soup	69
Pumpkin & Black Bean Soup	69
Stuffed Zucchini	70
Zucchini Lasagna	71
Stuffed Eggplant	72

Crusted Tilapia

Preheat oven to 400°

4 tilapia   1 tbl. parsley
¾ c. parmesan cheese   olive oil
2 tsp. paprika   salt & pepper

Directions:
Combine Parmesan cheese, paprika & parsley. Drizzle the fish
with olive oil and then sprinkle with the cheese mixture, salt &
pepper the top of each piece. Place on foil lined baking sheet and
broil for 10-12 minutes. Serve with lemon wedges. These are
soooo good!

Baked/Grilled Salmon

Preheat oven to 450° or grill, yum!

1 ½ lbs. salmon fillets   ⅓ c. honey
lemon pepper to taste   ⅓ c. water
garlic powder & salt to taste   ¼ cup olive oil
⅓ c. Braggs aminos (soy sauce)

Directions:
Season salmon fillets with lemon pepper, garlic powder and salt.
In small bowl stir together aminos, honey, water and oil. Place fish
in plastic bag with liquid mixture, seal and turn to coat. Refrigerate
for 2 hours or more. If grilling, lightly oil preheated grill, grill 6 to 8
minutes per side or until the fish flakes with fork. If baking, wrap
each fillet in tin foil, seal and bake for approx. 15 minutes, test with
fork for flakiness. Salmon is so very good for you!

54

Grilled Salmon w/Avocado Salsa

2 lbs. salmon cut in 4 pieces
1 tbl. virgin olive oil
1 tsp. sea salt
1 tsp. ground coriander
1 tsp.ground cumin
1 tsp. paprika powder
1 tsp. onion powder
1 tsp. pepper
3 tbl. virgin olive oil

Avocado Salsa:
1 avocado, sliced
1 sm. red onion, sliced
3 mild hot peppers,
    sliced
2 tbl. cilantro chopped
juice from 2 limes
salt & pepper to taste

Directions:
Mix the salt, coriander, cumin, paprika, onion and pepper together, rub into olive oiled salmon, refrigerate for 30 to 35 minutes. Meanwhile preheat the grill. Combine the avocado, onion, hot peppers, cilantro, lime juice, and salt & pepper in a bowl, mix well, chill until ready to use. Grill to desired doneness. Serve salmon topped with avocado salsa with rice as a side.

Baked Salmon

Preheat oven to 375º

2 salmon

2- 4 tbl. olive oil

2 lemons

garlic powder

salt & pepper

½ onion, sliced

Directions:

Place salmon on individual heavy duty oiled foil pieces large enough to cover and wrap completely around the salmon. Slice one lemon in halve and squeeze juice over salmon, slice the other lemon (4 or 5 slices) and place on top of salmon, sprinkle with garlic, salt and pepper. Top with sliced onions. Close foil around salmon so no juice leaks out. Bake for 10 to 13 minutes, till salmon flakes when separated with fork. Adapted from *Kim Halls* recipe.

Cauliflower Crust Pizza

Preheat oven to 450°

1 c. riced cauliflower
1 c. shredded mozzarella cheese
1 egg beaten
1 tsp. dried oregano

½ tsp. garlic, crushed
½ tsp. garlic powder
olive oil (optional)
pizza sauce

Directions:
Take cauliflower and run over grader until it is all riced. Place in glass bowl and microwave for 8 min. Spray cookie sheet or pizza pan with cooking spray. In bowl stir together cauliflower, cheese and egg. Add oregano, crushed garlic and garlic powder, stir. Pat into cookie sheet or pizza pan and brush olive oil over top to help with browning. Bake for 15 minutes. Add any toppings you would like, do a quick broil to warm the toppings. You'll be surprised!

Zesty Chicken Kabobs

Preheat the Grill!

3 tbl. Braggs Aminos
2 tbl. honey
1 tbl. sunflower oil
 Juice of 1 lime

1 tsp. garlic, minced
4 chicken breast
pineapple chunks
1 c. green, red, or yellow
   pepper

Directions:
In a small bowl combine aminos, honey, sunflower oil, lime juice and garlic. Cut chicken breasts into bite size pieces and place in soy sauce mixture, mix to coat each piece, refrigerator at least 30 minutes. Meanwhile, soak bamboo sticks in water for 5 minutes, cut peppers into bite size pieces. Place chicken, peppers and pineapple alternately on sticks and grill.

Honey Sauced Chicken

Preheat oven to 350° or Crock Pot

¾ lb. chicken breast
½ tsp. sea salt
¼ tsp. black pepper
½ c. honey
¼ tsp. red pepper flakes

¼ c. Braggs Aminos
⅛ c. onion, chopped
⅛ c. tomato sauce
1 clove garlic, minced
1 tbl. olive oil

Directions:

For Crock Pot: Season both sides of chicken with sea salt and pepper, put into crock pot. In a small bowl, combine pepper flakes, honey, Braggs Aminos, onion, tomato sauce, oil, garlic, pour over chicken and cook on low for 3 hrs. Cut chicken into bite size pieces, return to crock pot and mix with sauce. Serve over rice.

For baking: dice chicken and season all sides with sea salt and pepper, place in a 8 x 8 pan, pour sauce over chicken, bake for 20 minutes, stirring after 10 minutes. Serve over rice.

Loaded Chicken or Tuna Salad

2-3 c. shredded chicken or tuna
2 green onions
1 small red onion
1 red bell pepper, roasted
1 yellow bell pepper, roasted

2 stalks celery
1 carrot, shredded
1-2 avocados
salt & pepper to taste
½ c. Bolthouse farms
    dressing, ranch

Directions:
Chop green onion, red onion, bell peppers, celery. Peel and shred carrot. Cut avocado in half, remove pit with a spoon and scoop out the meat and chop. Mix together with dressing, season with salt & pepper and serve on fresh out of the oven Flax Seed Fococcia Bread (pg. 30). Bolthouse farm dressings do not have sugar or other ingredients you want to avoid. Choose your flavor, ranch is nice.

Roasted Chicken Salad w/Almonds

2 c. cubed cooked chicken
½ c. + sliced almonds
½ c. celery, chopped
½ c. dried cherries, chopped
1 6 oz. plain greek yogurt
½ brick cream cheese

1 tbl. lemon juice
1 tsp. poultry seasoning
1 tbs. Dijon mustard
1 tsp. sea salt
2 tsp. pepper

Directions:
Combine chicken, almonds, celery and dried cherries in a medium bowl. In another sm. bowl stir together yogurt, cream cheese, lemon juice, poultry seasoning, mustard and salt & pepper. Add to chicken mixture, toss gently. Serve on crisp lettuce leaves with almonds sprinkled on top. Cool and nutritious!

Thai Chicken

1 rotisserie chicken
1 13.5 oz can coconut milk
1 ½ or 2 tbl. of curry paste

4 tbl. honey
salt & pepper to taste
fresh basil leaves

Directions:
Pull meat from chicken in large pieces. Spoon 1 ½ to 2 tbl. of coconut milk into med. skillet over med. high heat. Stir in curry paste. Add honey, remaining coconut milk, salt and pepper. Bring to a simmer and taste, adjust with salt & pepper if needed. Add chicken, stir in fresh basil leaves and warm through. Serve over rice with lime wedges.

Chicken Tacos, Crock Pot

1 jar salsa (with no sugar)
1 tbl. taco seasoning

4 chicken breasts

Directions:
Put the entire jar of salsa in crock pot. Stir in taco seasoning, lay chicken breasts on top and cook on low overnight, 7 to 8 hours. Could this be any easier?

Honey Chicken, Crock Pot

1 c. pineapple juice
¾ c. honey

⅓ c. Braggs Aminos
2 lbs. chicken breast

Directions:
Mix liquid ingredients and place in crock pot. Lay chicken on top and cook on low for 6 to 8 hours. They will fall apart. This is great on rice or quinoa.

Coconut Chicken

2 lbs. boneless chicken breast
2 lg. eggs
¼ c. coconut milk
1 ½ c. almond flour

1 c. bread crumbs
1 c. shredded coconut
1 tsp. salt
½ c. olive oil

Directions:
Cut each breast into 6 even strips, ½ inch or less. In one bowl whisk together eggs and coconut milk until well combined. In another bowl combine flour & salt, in still another bowl mix bread crumbs and shredded coconut. Heat ¼ cup oil in a skillet until just below smoking. While oil is heating, dredge strips in each bowl in the order listed. Dip chicken in egg/milk mixture, then crumb mixture and last, in shredded coconut mixture. Place strips in pan but don't over crowd or the pan will cool. Fry strips 2 to 3 minutes on each side or until golden brown and crispy. Place on plate with paper towel to drain any excess. Serve with the dipping sauce of your choice!

61

Honey Lime Shrimp

½ lb. lg. shrimp, cleaned
¼ c. olive oil
2 tbl. honey
1 sm. lime, juice & zest

2 cloves garlic, smashed
½ tsp. sea salt
¼ tsp. pepper
¼ tsp. red pepper flakes

Directions:
Place all ingredients except shrimp in a large Ziploc bag, shake to mix, add shrimp, and squeeze as much air out as possible and close. Place in fridge for 30 to 60 minutes, flipping the bag twice to evenly coat shrimp. Take shrimp out of fridge and let sit for 10 minutes. Heat a large skillet over med-high heat; add shrimp (no need for oil) in one layer. Cook for one minute until they curl up and turn pink, flip for another 30 seconds or so until they are opaque.

Lemon Butter Shrimp

Preheat oven to 350°

1 pkg. shrimp, frozen, thawed
1 stick butter

1 lemon
italian seasoning

Directions:
Melt butter in shallow pan or cookie sheet, layer slices of lemon on top of butter. Place shrimp on top of lemon slices in one layer. Sprinkle Italian seasoning on top and bake for 15 minutes. Easy Breezy! And, oh so good.

Quinoa Burgers

2 rounded c. cooked quinoa
¾ c. cheese of choice
½ c. small curd cottage cheese
3 eggs
3 tbl. almond flour
olive oil for frying
1 med. carrot, finely grated (or shredded zucchini squeezed dry)

2 green onions
½ tsp. stevia
¼ tsp. pepper & cumin
⅛ tsp. sea salt
⅛ tsp. garlic powder

Directions:
Mix all ingredients except olive oil well with hands or fork. Make into patties and fry in hot olive oiled skillet until browned on both sides. Serve between Flax Seed Focaccia Bread slices (pg. 30).

Zucchini Pizza

Preheat oven to 400°

Sauce:

2 zucchini
1 sm. onion
1 green bell pepper
dill, graded cheese, oil

2 tomatoes, chopped
2-3 garlic cloves, graded
salt, pepper, thyme, curry
any other spices desired

Directions:
Slice zucchini lengthwise very thin. Place on oven tray, brush on oil. Mix all the *Sauce* ingredients and spread on zucchini slices. Arrange thin sliced peppers and onions on zucchini slices, sprinkle with cheese and dill. Sprinkle with other spices desired. Bake for about 25 minutes.

Taco Roll Ups

1 lb. ground turkey
1 tbl. taco seasoning
½ c. water
¾ c. shredded Mexican cheese blend
tortillas

1 16 oz. can refried beans
½ c. salsa
1 tsp. oregano
sour cream
guacamole

Directions:
Brown ground turkey in a large skillet over med. high heat, drain any fat. Add taco seasoning and water, stir and simmer for 3 minutes. For a smooth consistency you can pour the turkey into a blender with 4 or 5 short pulses to eliminate chunks. Heat a tortilla in the microwave for 10 seconds, spread with ½ c. of meat mixture, top with refried beans, salsa and cheese. Fold in the sides, roll up the tortilla. Tightly wrap in plastic wrap and refrigerate up to 24 hours. Cut in half at serving time after heating in Microwave. Or… serve immediately with sour cream and guacamole. Makes 6 roll ups.

Ratatouille

2 tbl. olive oil
1 lg. onion
4-5 big garlic cloves
1 sm. eggplant
1 red, yellow or orange pepper

1 zucchini
salt & pepper to taste
1 tsp. oregano
3 tomatoes, chopped
handful of spinach

Directions:
In a large skillet, heat olive oil over medium heat, sauté halved &
sliced onion until soft, add crushed garlic and sauté for one minute.
Chop eggplant into bite size pieces add to pan and cook another 5
minutes, add more oil if needed, until eggplant is soft. Chop
peppers and zucchini into small pieces, add to pan. Season with
salt & pepper. Cook for about 10 minutes until soft with golden
edges. Add oregano and tomatoes; cook until mixture is thick with
moisture cooked off. Add spinach until wilted, serve immediately.
Use any leftovers for pizza topping.

Sweet Potato Cauliflower Soup

Preheat oven to 400°

1 lg. head cauliflower
1 sweet onion, diced
3 med. sweet potatoes
2 cloves garlic

7 c. filtered water
olive oil for drizzling
salt to taste

Directions:
Cut cauliflower into bite sized pieces, place on ungreased cookie sheet, drizzle with olive oil. Roast in oven until golden brown (tender but not mushy) 20-30 minutes, let cool. Meanwhile, in large stockpot, bring diced onion, sweet potato, peeled and cut into 1" pieces, garlic and water to a boil, salt and stir. Reduce heat, keep at a constant simmer until sweet potatoes are tender, and add cauliflower. Divide soup into 2 parts. When cool, blend one part in blender until smooth, combine with second part and stir. Salt to taste, warm up on stove top if needed. Yum! So good when the leaves are swirling outside!

Tomato/Avocado Pizza

Preheat oven to 400°

1 Cauliflower Pizza Crust, pg. 56
2 avocados cut in 1" pieces
2 med. tomatoes, sliced & seeded
1 med. red onion, diced

1 ½ c. italian cheese
Pesto Sauce
Avocado Sauce
lemon juice

Directions:
Use the Cauliflower Pizza Crust recipe (pg. 56) for the crust and follow those directions. After you cut the avocados (cut them last) sprinkle with lemon juice so they won't turn brown. Spread the crust with Pesto (recipe in Dips & Spreads). Place avocados, tomatoes and onions on top of pesto. Sprinkle cheese on top and cook for about 10 minutes until the veggies are hot. Drizzle with Avocado Sauce (pg. 107) and enjoy!

Asparagus Soup

2 tbl. butter
1 sm. onion, chopped
1 stalk celery, chopped
pinch garlic powder

3 tbl. amaranth flour
2 c. chicken broth
1 lb. asparagus
salt & pepper to taste

Directions:
Cut asparagus in half and steam until soft, 7 to 10 minutes. In a 3 qt. sauce pot melt butter to sauté onion, celery and garlic powder over med. heat until onions are soft. Stir in flour and mix well. Add broth and milk stirring until boiling. When mixture thickens place in a blender with the asparagus (leaving some out for adding in later) and blend with the top or knob off since the food is hot. When smooth ad extra asparagus, salt & pepper to taste. So yummy!

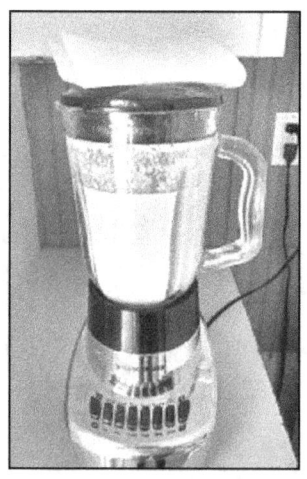

Asparagus Soup and the Blender I use!

Butternut Squash Soup

Preheat oven to 200°

1 butternut squash	1 tsp. garlic powder
1 can coconut milk	salt & pepper to taste

Directions:
Wash off squash and place in the oven whole for about two and a half hours, until the skin is darker and soft to the touch. Cut squash in half, scoop out seeds, scoop out meat and place in bowl. Add the coconut milk, garlic powder and salt & pepper; blend with immersion blender until smooth. If you like your soup less thick, add a little almond milk or flax milk to desired consistency. Enjoy!

Pumpkin & Black Bean Soup

1 onion, diced	1 32 oz. can pumpkin puree
4 c. chicken or veggie stock	½ tsp. curry powder
1 14 oz. can diced tomatoes	½ tsp. cinnamon
1 15 oz. black beans, rinsed	¾ tsp. cayenne pepper
salt & pepper to taste	

Directions:
In soup pot heat oil over med. heat, add onions when hot and sauté for 5 minutes till clear. Add broth, tomatoes, beans and pumpkin; bring to a boil, stirring so soup does not burn on the bottom. Reduce heat to medium low and add spices, simmer 5 minutes.

Stuffed Zucchini

Preheat oven to 400°

2 zucchini
1 onion
½ tomato
¼ tsp. curry powder

4 slices bacon, crisp
1 tbl. sour cream
1 tsp. thyme
salt & pepper to taste

Directions:
Slice zucchini in half lengthwise, spoon out the meat leaving about a ¼ to ½ inch sides. Chop the zucchini meat, onion and tomato. Sauté the onions in a little oil, add the curry powder when almost done. Add all the rest of the ingredients including the zucchini meat, cook for a few minutes. Place mixture in the zucchini boats, place in a baking dish and bake for about 20 minutes. You can put them in the broiler when their done to brown the top. Sprinkle with fresh parsley and a little cheese if you want.

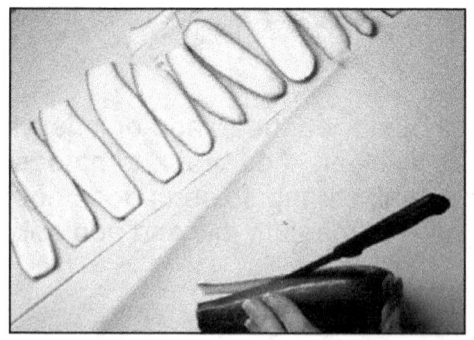

Cutting and Sweating Zucchini for *Zucchini Lasagna*

Zucchini Lasagna

Preheat oven to 350°

2 zucchini
1 lb. ground beef
3 cloves garlic
½ onion, chopped
2 tbl. basil
1 lg. chopped tomato
1 lg. can italian tomatoes

15 oz. ricotta cheese
¼ c. parmesan cheese
15 oz. monterey jack
1 lg. egg
1 tsp. olive oil
salt & pepper

Directions:
Slice zucchini very thin lengthwise. I cut off the skin, but you don't have. Place slices on parchment paper and sprinkle with salt to sweat the zucchini. I let it set for 2 hours or so, this gets most of the water out. Meanwhile, fry ground beef, drain, add garlic, onion, basil, chopped tomato and italian tomatoes and cook until thick, 10 min. or so. Pat zucchini with a paper towel to soak up the water and fry slices in a pan with olive oil to cook through. This takes 30 seconds or so, they cook quickly. Mix the cheeses together with egg and salt & pepper. Now building the dish, in a deep pan place a spoonful of meat sauce on the bottom, lay zucchini on top, sprinkle some cheese mixture on top, spoon some meat sauce on top of that. Continue layering until all the zucchini is gone and finish with cheese and sauce. Cook for 20 to 30 minutes. One of my family's favorite!

Stuffed Eggplant

Preheat oven to 350°

2 lg. firm eggplant
2 tbl. olive oil
1 med. onion, chopped
4 cloves garlic, diced
1 c. green & red pepper, chopped

1 14 oz. can diced tomatoes
¾ c. quinoa, cooked
½ tsp. salt and ¼ tsp. pepper
½ c. shredded Italian blend

Directions:
Cut eggplant in halve lengthwise from top to bottom. Scoop out the pulp to within ¼ inch of the skin, careful, don't break the skin. Chop pulp into ½ inch pieces and set aside. Place both halves in microwave dish with 2 tbl. of water. Cover with plastic wrap and microwave for 5 min. In a fry pan sauté onion, garlic and peppers in olive oil until onion is shiny and soft, about 5 minutes. Add eggplant pulp and continue cooking another 5 minutes or so, till eggplant is no longer white but shiny. Add tomatoes, cooked quinoa, salt and pepper and cook till everything is heated. Fill the softened eggplant boats with mixture. Any leftover can be used as a side dish or piled on top of the boats. Sprinkle with cheese and enjoy. This recipe is courtesy of my sister, *Sonie Curtis!*

Notes

Notes

Desserts

Apple Crisp	76
Easy Apple Oatmeal Bars	77
Apple Crisp, Crock Pot	78
No Bake Apple Walnut Tart	78
Frozen Chocolate Banana Bites	79
Banana Raspberry Ice Cream	79
Frozen Yogurt Bananas	80
Chocolate Beet Cake	80
Brownies w/ Cherries & Ganache	81
Brownies, Garbanzo Beans	82
Carmel	83
Cookie Dough Balls	83
Dessert Crepes	84
Fresh Fruit Cobbler Roll-ups	85
Gingerbread Cookies	85
Greek Yogurt Parfait	86
Healthy Frozen Yogurt	86
Key Lime Pie	87
No Bake Energy Bites	88
No Bake Coconut Cream Cheese Balls	88
Pumpkin Pie Muffins	89
Pumpkin Cookies	89
Watermelon Cantaloupe Dessert	90

Apple Crisp

Preheat oven to 375º

⅓ c. almond flour
2 tbl. Stevia
⅓ c. regular oats
½ tsp. cinnamon
¼ tsp. chilled butter

3 tbl. walnuts, chopped
7 c. red apples, sliced
2 tbl. ground flax seed
¼ c. pure maple syrup

Directions:
Combine flour, Stevia, oats and ¼ tsp. cinnamon in a medium bowl, cut in butter with a knife or pastry blender until mixture is crumbly, stir in walnuts. Combine apples and remaining ingredients in a separate bowl, toss well. Place apple mixture into an 8-inch square baking dish or 1 ½ quart greased casserole, sprinkle with crumb mixture and bake for 45 minutes or until golden brown and apples are tender. I like it with a dollop of sour cream on top.

Easy Apple Oatmeal Bars

Preheat oven to 350°

2 c. unsweetened almond milk
½ c. pecans, chopped
½ c. ground flax seed
1 ½ tsp. ground cinnamon

1 ½ c. oats
½ c. raisins
2 tsp. vanilla extract
2 apples, cored & grated

Directions:
Mix all ingredients together in a large bowl one at a time stirring while adding. Transfer to a foil or parchment paper lined 9 x 13 baking pan, press down and smooth out the top. Bake until firm and golden brown, about 1 hour. Let cool in pan, cut into squares, serve warm or at room temperature. Good with whipped whole cream and drizzled with honey!

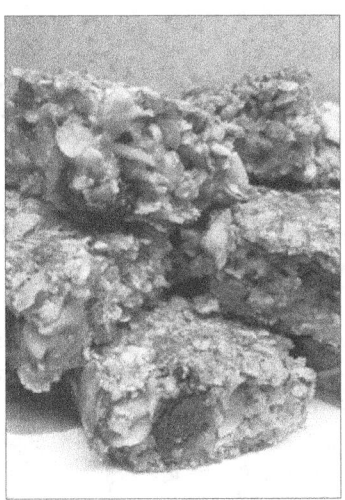

Easy Apple Oatmeal Bars

Apple Crisp, Crock Pot

9 smallish apples
¼ c. butter
⅓ c. honey

¼ c. orange juice
2 tbl. vanilla
1 c. oatmeal for crumb top

Directions:
Chop up apples and place in bottom of crock pot. Toss the apples with cubed butter, honey, orange juice and vanilla. Cook on high for 3 hours. Mix oatmeal and coconut sugar, sprinkle on top of apples and place crock in oven on bottom rack for 5 to 7 minutes to crisp the topping, if desired. Or just sprinkle oatmeal mixture on top and enjoy!

No Bake Apple Walnut Tart

2 ½ c. walnuts   ½ tsp. salt   1 ½ c. dates

Filling:
3 green apples
juice of 1 lemon in 2 c. water
½ c. apple juice
¼ tsp. cinnamon

½ tsp. allspice
⅛ tsp. ground clove
2 tlb. honey
¼ c. raisins

Directions:
Combine walnuts, salt and dates (remove pits & cut stem end off if needed) in food processor or blender until well mixed but not smooth. Press evenly into a 9 inch tart pan. *Filling*: cut apples crosswise in ¼ inch thick slices, place in lemon water as your cutting. Put apples in a large skillet with the rest of ingredients and cook for 10 minutes, stirring frequently on med. heat. Remove apples from pan and cool. Continue cooking liquid till reduced to about half making a syrup and cool. Spread apples evenly over date crust. Brush apple syrup over apples. Serve with a dapple of Greek yogurt!

Frozen Chocolate Banana Bites

1 square unsweetened baking chocolate   1 c. Xylitol
½ stick butter   3 bananas

Directions:
Melt chocolate square & butter in a pan, add Xylitol, mix well till dissolved. Slice the bananas into bite size pieces while mixture is melting. When mixture is done, take off heat and drop 5 or so banana bites into chocolate mixture, coat and place on plate or wax paper. Put in freezer.
For a different twist, after slicing bananas, sandwich almond butter between 2 slices and freeze until ready to dip in chocolate. A great kid treat!

Banana Raspberry Ice Cream

2 frozen bananas cut in ½" slices   2 tbl. almond milk
½ c. frozen raspberries   ½ tsp. vanilla

Directions:
Place cut bananas on a plate to freeze for 2 or more hours. Place bananas and raspberries in a food processor or blender until well blended, add milk and vanilla, blend. You can eat it now as a soft serve or freeze for scooped ice cream. If you don't like raspberries you can substitute strawberries or blueberries or any other berry.

Frozen Yogurt Bananas

2 bananas
½ c. greek yogurt
1 tsp. cinnamon

½ c. crushed almonds or pecans
popsicle sticks

Directions:
Line a tray with parchment paper. Mix the yogurt and cinnamon and place on a plate. Place crushed almonds on another plate. Peel bananas, cut off one end and insert a popsicle stick. Roll the bananas in yogurt and then in almonds. Place on parchment paper and freeze about 45 minutes. Bananas will be creamy and firm but not completely frozen.

Chocolate Beet Cake

Preheat oven to 350º

1 ¾ c. beets, 3 or 4 beet bulbs
3 eggs
1 ½ c. unrefined coconut sugar
1 tsp. vanilla
¾ c. coconut oil

¼ c. baking cocoa
2 c. amaranth flour
1 ½ tsp. baking soda
½ tsp. sea salt

Directions:
Steam beets until soft, about 15 min., puree in a blender or food processor, add eggs, sugar, vanilla and oil, blend until smooth. Add cocoa and other dry ingredients mixing with a spoon. Pour into a 9 x 13 greased pan. Cook for 30 minutes, until knife or tooth pick comes out clean. Really delicious!

Brownies with Berries & Ganache

Preheat oven to 350°

4 oz. unsweetened chocolate squares, chopped
1 lg. avocado, mashed
3 tbl. honey
¼ c. dried cherries, chopped
1 tbl. vanilla

1 egg
1 tbl. almond milk
pinch of salt

Frosting:
¼ c. coconut milk
¼ c. cocoa powder

¾ c. honey

Directions:
In a small, microwave-safe bowl, melt the chocolate for 10 second intervals, stirring between each interval. Pour melted chocolate into a food processor or blender and add the avocado, honey, vanilla, egg and a pinch of salt. Blend until smooth making sure there are no lumps. Transfer mixture to a medium bowl and add the chopped cherries. Fill greased muffin tins about ¾ of the way up and bake until they pull away from the sides, about 25 - 30 minutes. Let brownies cool in the tin for 5 minutes and then using a knife lift them out onto a cooling rack. Now, heat the coconut milk and honey on medium heat until just about boiling. Remove from heat and add the cocoa powder, whisk until blended. Spoon the ganache on a medium plate with sides and dunk brownies into the frosting, place back on rack. Let cool and DEVOUR

Brownies, Garbanzo Bean

Preheat oven to 325°

1 ½ c. garbanzo beans (about one can) rinsed, drained
½ c. turbinado sugar   2 tsp. vanilla
¼ c. cocoa powder   2 eggs
½ tsp. baking powder   1 tbl. coconut oil

Directions:
Place ingredients in a food chopper, I use the one below, in the
order listed. Chop until well blended. Place in a 9 x 9 parchment
paper lined cake pan. Cook for 20 minutes or so, until a knife
inserted comes out clean. These are so good and you won't know
the difference between a box mix and these brownies.

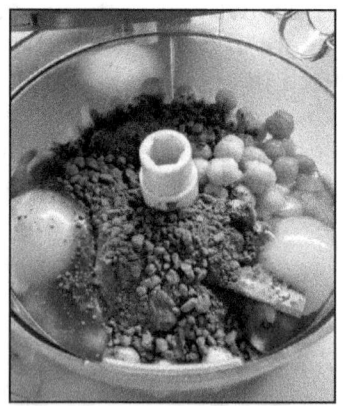

Brownies, Garbanzo Bean
The Food Chopper I use

Caramel

1 ½ c. honey   ¾ tsp. sea salt
1 ¾ c. heavy cream

Directions:
Put honey in a saucepan and bring to a simmer (it will bubble around the edges). Mix heavy cream & salt together, add this mixture to the honey and bring to a boil. Once it boils, lower the heat and keep an active simmer going. When it begins to darken in color it is done (about 13 minutes). Take off burner and let cool at room temperature. Caramel that is NOT with sugar! Dip apples or any fruit in caramel.

Cookie Dough Balls

2 ½ c. almond flour   1 tbl. vanilla
3 tbl. coconut flour   ½ c. pecan bits
10 tsp. softened butter   2 bars unsweetened
⅓ c. honey   chocolate

Directions:
Cream together 8 tsp. softened butter, honey and vanilla. Stir in almond flour and coconut flour. Batter will be stiff enough to form into balls but not too dry. Add pecan bits and form into balls, refrigerate on parchment covered cookie sheet for 30 minutes. Melt chocolate in a sauce pan; add the remaining 2 tsp. of butter and a little honey. When melted, remove balls from fridge and roll in chocolate. Place back on cookie sheet and refrigerate for another 30 minutes. Enjoy!

Dessert Crepes

3 parts old fashioned oats   water
1 part sunflower seeds   cream cheese
1 egg   desired fruit
olive oil   honey

Directions:
Grind oats and seeds in a coffee grinder. The size of the grinder will determine the amounts used. My grinder is small so I use ¼ c. plus 1 tbl. of oats and 1 heaping tbl. of sunflower seeds. Place in a bowl and mix in egg. Add water to make crepe mix consistency. Mixture will be soup like. As you let the mixture set it will thicken. Just add a little water to keep the right consistency. Place 1 tsp. or less of oil on a paper towel and rub fry pan so there are no puddles. Pour in mix to coat pan thinly, fry on low until the sides start to crisp and the crepe can be flipped. Flip. Cook until you can lift the crepe with your hand. Place on plate and spread with softened cream cheese. I heat frozen blueberries and strawberries in the microwave and pour them on the crepe, fold it in half and drizzle with honey. This is my husband's favorite dessert!

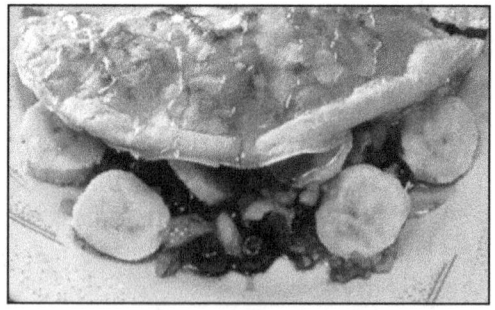

Dessert Crepe

Fresh Fruit Cobbler Roll Ups

Preheat oven to 140°

2 c. sliced peaches or fruit of choice   2 tbl. honey
oil spray

Directions:
Puree sliced fruit in a blender with honey, pour into a nonstick
baking sheet coated with oil spray. Dry in oven until fruit peels
away easily from baking sheet. Store by rolling on plastic wrap
and keeping in a covered container in the refrigerator.

Gingerbread Cookies

Preheat oven to 350°

3 c. almond flour   3 tbl. ginger
3 c. date sugar   1 tbl. cinnamon
5 eggs   ½ tsp. ground cloves
1 tsp. sea salt   dried currants
½ tsp. nutmeg

Directions:
Mix almond flour, date sugar, eggs, sea salt, nutmeg, ginger,
cinnamon, and cloves until they form a solid lump of dough. Flour
a working surface and rolling pin, spread dough onto work surface
and roll until about ¼ inch thick. Cut shapes with a cookie cutter,
decorate with currants and place on parchment lined baking sheet,
bake until fragrant and slightly browned at the edges, 12 to 15
minutes. Cool on rack. *Merry Christmas!*

Greek Yogurt Parfait

1 c. fresh berries, 2 or 3 kinds
½ c. greek plain yogurt
½ oz. chopped almonds

1 tbl. cocoa nibs
or chopped cocoa chips
½ tbl. honey

Directions:
Alternate placing ingredients in a parfait cup in order until you are out of stuff with a dollop of yogurt on top. A fresh mint leaf looks pretty. Or sprinkle coconut flakes on top. Make up a few for quick breakfasts!

Healthy Frozen Yogurt

4 c. frozen strawberries
3 tbl honey

½ c. greek yogurt
1 tbl. lemon juice

Directions for *cake*:
Place all ingredients in the order listed into a food processor or blender. Mix until creamy and serve. Or place in a freezer container and freeze until you're ready to enjoy! Great on a hot summer day when your desiring ice cream but want something healthy.

Key Lime Pie

Crust:
¾ c. walnuts   ¾ c. dates
1½ tbl. cocoa powder   pinch sea salt

Filling:
1 ½ lg. avocados, peeled, cored   1 ½ bananas, peeled
¼ c. lime juice   1 tsp. vanilla
10 drops vanilla   stevia or honey to taste
⅓ c. coconut oil, melted

Directions:
Place nuts in a food processor or blender until finely ground, add in, cocoa powder, the dates and salt until mixture is broken down and sticks together. Press into a greased 8 inch spring-form pan and put into the fridge while making filling. Place all filling ingredients, except coconut oil, into a food processor and blend until smooth. Melt coconut oil and while the food processor is running, pour it in and process until well incorporated. Pour into the pan and spread evenly over crust. Cover and place in fridge for 3 or more hours until firm. You can garnish with coconut flakes, or fruit.

No Bake Energy Bites

1 c. oatmeal
½ c. nut butter
⅓ c. honey
1 c. coconut flakes

½ c. ground flax seed
½ c. mini chocolate chips
1 tsp. vanilla

Directions:
Mix everything above in a medium bowl until thoroughly incorporated, let chill in the refrigerator for half an hour. Roll into balls and enjoy! Store in an airtight container in fridge, will keep up to one week. Nice munchies on the go!

No Bake Coconut Cream Cheese Balls

1 8 oz. pkg cream cheese
1 can crushed pineapple, drained

1 c. pecans, chopped
3 c. flaked coconut

Directions:
Mix softened cream cheese and *well drained* pineapple until combined, fold in the pecans. Cover and refrigerate for 1 hour. Take out of refrigerator and roll into 1 inch balls, then roll balls in the coconut, refrigerate for 4 hours or overnight.

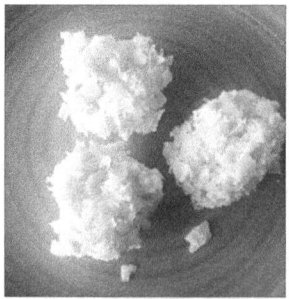

No Bake Coconut Cream Cheese Balls

Pumpkin Pie Muffins

Preheat oven to 350°

1½ c. almond flour
¼ tsp. sea salt
½ tsp. baking soda
1 tsp. cinnamon
½ tsp. nutmeg
pureed
¼ tsp. ginger

1 pinch ground cloves
2 tbl. olive oil
½ c. agave nectar
2 large eggs
1 c. fresh pumpkin

Directions:
Combine first seven ingredients in a bowl. Mix in a blender oil, agave, eggs and pumpkin until smooth. Stir wet ingredients into dry, scoop into paper muffin pan liners, bake for 40 to 45 minutes. Cool and enjoy with whipped whole cream sweetened with Turbinado sugar.

Pumpkin Cookies

Preheat oven to 350°

1 ½ c. pumpkin puree
1 ½ c. almond flour
¼ c. softened butter
¼ c. coconut oil
½ tsp. sea salt

¾ c. honey or agave nectar
1 egg
1 tbl. pumpkin pie spice
1 tsp. baking soda

Directions:
Process all ingredients in a food processor until smooth. Form ping pong ball size balls and place on cookie sheets lined with parchment paper. Bake for about 20 minutes. After 5 min. in the oven, press down each cookie with a fork and finish baking. Cool and serve.

Watermelon Cantaloupe Dessert

2 c. cantaloupe, 1" cubes
1 lb. strawberries, hulled
2 c. seedless watermelon, 1" cubes
1 tbl. fresh lime juice
1 cucumber, peeled, seeded, chopped

Directions:
Place cantaloupe, watermelon, cucumber, half the strawberries and lime juice in food processor or blender and puree. Chop remaining strawberries and stir into the mixture. Refrigerate until chilled. Refreshing!

Notes

Notes

Snacks

Apple Rings, Deep Fried   94
Chocolate Almonds   95
Cinnamon Roasted Almonds   95
Carrot Chips-Yeah...really!   96
Frozen Monster Pops   96
Granola Bars   97
Kale Chips   98
No-Bake Energy Bites   99
Pumpkin Pie Almonds   99
Sesame Truffles   100

Apple Rings, Deep Fried

1 c. amaranth flour
¼ tsp. baking powder
¼ tsp. salt
¼ tsp. cinnamon
1 lg. beaten egg

1 c. almond milk
4 lg. apples
olive oil for frying
cinnamon for sprinkling
honey for drizzling

Directions:
Add the first 4 ingredients together and mix. Add the egg and milk, mix well, set aside. Place olive oil in fry pan, about an inch or so deep. Turn fire on med. Slice the apples one at a time to avoid browning, about ¼ inch thick, cut out the centers. The oil should be ready now, drop 2 or 3 apple rings in the oil for about 2 minutes flipping once for 30 seconds or so until golden. You can start cutting the next apple. Place done apple rings on a paper plate with paper towel on top. Sprinkle with cinnamon and drizzle with honey. These are a bit messy but so good and fun for kids! It's like making healthy doughnuts!

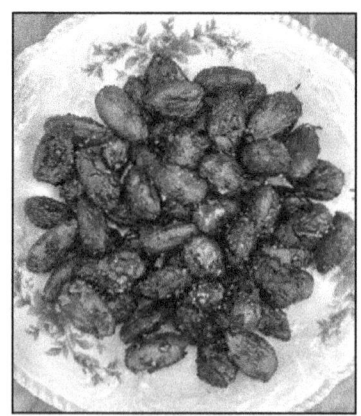

Chocolate Almonds

94

Chocolate Almonds

Preheat oven to 250°

2 c. raw almonds
1 tbl. coconut oil
2 tbl. date or rice syrup

1 tbl. cocoa powder
¼ tsp. sea salt
water

Directions:
Soak the almonds in water just to cover overnight, drain in the morning and air dry. Mix all remaining ingredients well, stir in nuts. Place them on parchment paper on a cookie sheet and bake for about an hour to an hour and a half, till no longer sticky/wet.

Cinnamon Roasted Almonds

Preheat oven to 325°

⅓ c. butter
2 egg whites
pinch of sea salt

1 c. Xylitol
3 c. soaked almonds
4 tsp. cinnamon

Directions:
In 13"x9" pan melt butter in oven about 7 min. Meanwhile, beat egg whites with salt until frothy; gradually add Xylitol beating to stiff peaks. Gently fold in almonds and cinnamon, pour mixture onto pan, toss with butter. Bake about 40 minutes, tossing every 10 minutes until almonds are crisp. Serve warm. Store cooled almonds in airtight container up to 2 weeks.

Carrot Chips – Yeah... really!

Preheat oven to 350°

carrots, as many as you want   cinnamon, sea salt, olive oil

Directions:
Peel with a potato peeler making thin carrots slices. Toss slices in olive oil and salt, or olive oil and cinnamon. Bake for 12 minutes. Cool and enjoy!

Frozen Monster Pops

1 c. baby spinach, packed tightly
2 med. ripe bananas
2 c. fresh pineapple
½ c. freshly squeezed orange juice (about 2 Valencia)

Directions:
Place ingredients in a blender in order listed and blend until smooth; you may have to scrape the sides. Pour into popsicle molds and freeze for 4 hours. The mixture will sweeten up when frozen. Kids will love these!

Granola Bars

Preheat oven to 250°

3 ½ c. rolled steel oats
1 c. raw sliced almonds
1 c. raw cashew pieces, or pecans
1 c. unsweetened shredded coconut
½ c. raw sunflower & pumpkin seeds
2 tsp. vanilla extract

½ tsp. ground nutmeg
2 tsp. ground cinnamon
1 ½ tsp. ground ginger
½ c. honey
¼ c. butter

Directions:
Cover baking sheet with parchment paper. Mix dry oats, almonds, cashews, coconut, seeds and spices together in a large bowl. Heat butter and honey in small saucepan over low heat till melted, stir in vanilla. Pour the hot liquids over the dry ingredients and stir together with rubber spatula until evenly coated. Spread onto parchment papered pan, bake for 75 minutes. Mixture will crisp as it cools. Half way to being cooled, press cut lines for bars with a butter knife. When cool, break the bars apart.

Kale Chips

Preheat oven to 275°

20 kale leaves
2 tbl. olive oil
½ tsp. salt & pepper

½ tsp. garlic powder
2 tsp. Italian herbs

Directions:
Wash kale leaves, dry with paper towel. In a large plastic bag place olive oil, salt & pepper, garlic powder and Italian herbs, drop in 10 leaves at a time and shake till well covered. Place on cookie sheet, not touching or overlapping, lined with parchment paper. Cook for 10 minutes or until crisp. These are soooo good!

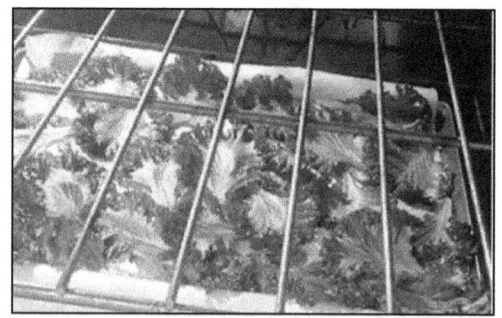

Kale Chips, ready to cook

No Bake Energy Bites

1 c. old-fashioned oatmeal
½ c. unsweetened chocolate chips
¼ c. toasted coconut flakes
½ c. flaxseed, ground

⅓ c. honey
1 tsp. vanilla
½ c. almond butter

Directions:
Stir all ingredients together in a med. bowl until mixed, let chill in the fridge for ½ hour. Then roll into balls, about 1" in diameter. Store in an airtight container, refrigerate up to one week. Makes about 20-25.

Pumpkin Pie Almonds

Preheat oven to 320º

2 c. soaked almonds
3 tsp. cinnamon
3 tsp. pumpkin pie spice

4 tbl. honey
1 tsp. vanilla
salt, pinch

Directions:
Mix all ingredients but almonds together, add almonds, bake for 20 minutes. Snack away!

Sesame Truffles

½ c. raw cashews
2 ¼ c. tahini, roasted or raw
¼ c. sesame seeds, raw or roasted

1 tsp. vanilla extract
¼ c. honey

Directions:
Tahini is a paste made from ground, hulled sesame seeds. You can buy it at Meijer and health food stores. Pulse cashews in food processor or blender until a coarse texture, add tahini, honey & vanilla, pulse until smooth. Place mixture in a bowl, refrigerate 2 hours. Then roll into1 inch balls, coat with sesame seeds. Keep refrigerated.

Notes

Notes

Dips & Spreads

Spinach/Artichoke Dip	104
Apricot Spread	104
Bean Dip, So Simple!	105
Debra's Tortilla Chips	105
Chocolate Dip	106
Cookie Dough Dip	106
Hawaiian Dip	107
Onion Chutney	107
Pesto	108
Apple Chutney	108
Crock Pot Apple Butter	109
Avocado Sauce	109
Hummus	110
Avocado Hummus	110
Mayonnaise	110
Raspberry Chipotle Sauce	111
Basic Red Salsa	111

Spinach Artichoke Dip

Preheat oven to 350°

4 oz. softened cream cheese
¼ c. sour cream
⅛ c. whole cream
1 tsp. pepper, garlic powder, salt to your liking
1 10 oz. box frozen chopped spinach, thawed
1 14 oz. can artichoke hearts, drained & roughly chopped
1 c. shredded parmesan-romano cheese mix

Directions:
Combine first 3 ingredients thoroughly in a bowl. Add the remaining ingredients one at a time as listed & spread mixture into 8x8 baking dish. Bake for 25-30 minutes or until bubbling & melted.

Apricot Spread

3 carrots chopped
1 c. raw cashew pieces, divided
15 dried apricots quartered, about ½ cup

Directions:
Bring carrots to boil in enough water to cover, reduce heat to med. low, cover & simmer until tender, 10 minutes or so. Add ¾ c. cashews & apricots, cover and continue to simmer until carrots are very soft, 5 to 7 minutes. Saving ½ cup of the cooking water, drain ingredients well. Puree reserved water and mixture in food processor or blender until smooth. Chill 1 hour, spread on your homemade flat bread.

Bean Dip, So Simple

1 can northern beans
garlic powder,
salt & pepper to taste

Directions:
Rinse beans and puree with garlic powder, salt & pepper with a hand blender. That's it! Use as a veggie dip. You can use black beans, white beans and vary the spices to your liking. They really are so good with homemade chips.

Debra's Tortilla Chips

2 lg. corn tortillas   2 tbl. olive oil   salt

Directions:
Oil both sides of tortillas. Cut in chip size pieces with a pizza slicer and place on a cookie sheet. Sprinkle with salt. Cook at 250° for about 10 minutes, until the chips are crisp. Easy, quick!

Chocolate Dip

3 ripe avocados
¼ c. cocoa powder
½ c. honey
pinch of salt

Directions:
Cut avocados in half, remove pit and scoop out the meat. Place meat in a food processor along with honey, cocoa powder and a pinch of salt. Pulse until well blended. If you use a blender, add a little almond milk until well blended, maybe a tbl. or so. The blender needs a little more liquid than the food processor. GREAT with fresh fruit! Your guest won't know its avocado!

Cookie Dough Dip

1 can drained chickpeas
⅛ tsp. sea salt
½ tsp. vanilla extract
⅓ c. unsweetened chocolate chips

¼ c. almond butter
¼ c. almond milk
3 tbl. maple syrup
2 tsp. vanilla

Directions:
Discard loose skins from chickpeas and rinse, add all ingredients except chocolate chips together in a blender or food processor until smooth, hand mix in chocolate chips. Good veggie dip for kids!

Hawaiian Dip

8 oz. cream cheese, softened
20 oz. can crushed/chunk pineapple
2½ c. coconut
nuts or cherries to top dip with

Directions:
Blend all ingredients together in food processor to crush pineapple and coconut pieces. Refrigerate at least 30 minutes before serving. Good with pita crackers, or celery. Great summer recipe!

Onion Chutney

This chutney is a good dip for veggies or homemade chips.

2 tbl. olive oil
2 tsp. cumin seeds
1 tsp. mustard seeds
4 dried green chilies, crushed
6 c. onions, sliced

2 tsp. chili powder
1 tsp. salt
¼ c. lemon juice
¼ c. Stevia or Xylitol

Directions:
Heat oil in pan, add cumin, mustard seeds, and dried chilies, heat until they sputter. Add onions and sauté until golden brown. Add chili powder, salt, lemon juice & Stevia or Xylitol & bring to a boil for 1 minute. Remove from heat and seal in sterilized jars.

Pesto

3 tsp. white vinegar
1 tsp. balsamic vinegar
½ tsp. lemon juice
½ tsp. honey
¼ tsp. paprika
½ c. cashews, chopped

2 cloves garlic
2 green onions, chopped
1 tsp pepper
1 tsp. ground cumin
½ c. fresh cilantro, chopped
¼ c. olive oil

Directions:
Put everything in a blender until mixed well.

Apple Chutney

1 lb. apples, peeled, cored, cut in small pieces
1 sm. onion, diced
1 jalapeno pepper, diced and seeds removed
1 tbl. garlic, chopped
1 c. Xylitol or honey
1 c. apple cider vinegar
½ c. raisins
½ tsp. ground turmeric, cinnamon, cayenne
¼ tsp. ground ginger, allspice, cloves

Directions:
Put everything in a large saucepan, cook until boiling, reduce heat and simmer until it thickens, about 45-60 minutes. Easy! Enjoy with pork chops or on turkey, or anything you would like!

Crock Pot Apple Butter

10 med. apples, Red Delicious
2 c. unsweetened apple juice
¼ c. water
¼ c. Braggs apple cider vinegar
1 tbl. cinnamon

½ tsp. pure vanilla
¼ tsp. ground cloves
¼ tsp. ground nutmeg
pinch of sea salt

Directions:
Place cored and sliced apples (not peeled) into a large crock pot, pour apple juice on top. Add water, apple cider vinegar and spices, stir all ingredients together and cover. Cook for 15 hours on low. The liquid will reduce and the apples will be very soft, dark in color and smell GREAT. Turn the crock pot off and let the apples cook for 30 minutes or so, then transfer mixture to a blender or use an immersion blender and blend until completely smooth. Let the mixture cool, then place into storage containers. Stores in the fridge for about three weeks. Or, place in ½ pint freezer-safe canning jars, put the lid on and let cool. Place into freezer for six months and you have homemade *Christmas Gifts*!

Avocado Sauce

½ c. mayo (pg. 108)
½ c. sour cream
2 tbl. almond milk
1 green onion, roughly chopped
2 cloves garlic

½ c. cilantro, chopped
1 avocado
1 lemon, the juice
salt & pepper to taste

Directions:
Put everything in a blender until mixed well, scraping as you go.

Hummus

1 can garbanzo beans   1 tsp. pepper & salt
1 tsp. garlic powder

Directions:
Blend all ingredients together in food processor or blender till smooth And... that's it! You can add chopped tomatoes on top or anything you want. I LOVE this dip and make it all the time!

Avocado Hummus

1 can garbanzo beans   1 tsp. pepper & salt
2 avocados, scoop out meat   1 tsp. garlic powder

Directions:
Blend all ingredients together in food processor or blender. Enjoy!

Mayonnaise

4 egg yolks   ⅔ c. olive oil
1 tbl. lemon juice   ⅔ c. coconut oil
1 tsp. dijon mustard   salt & pepper

Directions:
Wisk egg yolks until smooth, add lemon juice, mustard and spices, mix well. Starting with olive oil, add a little at a time while whisking until it starts to emulsify, keep adding until all oil is incorporated. Store in the fridge up to one week.

110

Raspberry Chipotle Sauce

½ c. red onion, chopped
2 tbl. olive oil
2 garlic cloves, minced
1 ½ lg. chipotle peppers minced (from a can in adobe sauce)
2 pints raspberries

15 oz. can tomato sauce
¼ c. + 2 tsp. honey
¼ c. apple cider vinegar

Directions:
Heat a lg. sauté pan to med. high, add oil and onion, sauté for 2-3 minutes until onions are translucent. Add garlic cloves and chipotle peppers, stir for 30 seconds. Add tomato sauce, honey, apple cider vinegar, stir until mixed. Add raspberries, stir till boiling and reduce heat to simmer for 10-15 minutes, stirring often. Remove from heat and cool. Store in an airtight container in the fridge.

Basic Red Salsa

4 med. tomatoes, finely chopped
1 can tomato sauce
3 green chilies, mild or hot, diced
3 green onions, chopped
1 garlic clove, crushed

¼ tsp. oregano
¼ tsp ground cumin.
¼ tsp. chili powder
salt & pepper to taste

Directions:
In order listed combine all ingredients in glass bowl. Cover and refrigerate. For best results make the day before serving. Love salsa!

Notes

Smoothies

Brain Boost Blueberry Dream   114
Breakfast Smoothie   114
Carrot Cooler   115
Green Almond Smoothie   115
Choco Raspberry Smoothie   115
Dessert in a Glass   116
Dreamy Mango Smoothie   116
My Morning Smoothie   117
Strawberry-Peach Smoothie   118
South American Quinoa Drink   118
Watermelon Breeze   119
Frozen Smoothie Bags   119

Liquid for Smoothies

To reduce thickness of smoothie I add purified or distilled water. You can also use almond milk, flax seed milk, rice milk, carrot juice, and unsweetened apple juice, goat milk... anything healthy and without sugars. Cow's milk is not recommended due to lactose allergies. The less liquid you use the thicker the smoothie will be.

Brain Boost Blueberry Dream

1 c. blueberries, frozen semi thawed
1 tsp. flax seed oil, cold-pressed
1 sm. banana

Directions:
Combine all the ingredients in a blender and process until smooth.

Breakfast Smoothie

⅓ c. almonds
2 bananas
½ c. cooked oatmeal, cooled
syrup

⅓ c. greek yogurt
1 tbl. honey
1 tbl. maple

Directions:
Soak almonds overnight to soften and sprout. Drain almonds in the morning. Combine all ingredients in a blender until smooth. A sweet drink!

Carrot Cooler

3 bags of frozen shredded carrot
3 to 4 tangerines, peeled
1 sm. Fuji apple, cored

1 ½ c. green grapes
3 stalks of celery

Directions:
Combine all ingredients in a blender until smooth. Carrots won't
turn to juice easily unless they are frozen. You can put all the
ingredients in a juicer, but most juicers leave a lot of pulp and you
want all the nutrients you can get.

Green Almond Smoothie

½ c. almond milk
2 tbl. almond butter, no sugar

1 sm. banana
1 sm. kale leaves,
10 or 15

Directions:
Combine all ingredients in a blender and process until smooth.

Choco Raspberry Smoothie

½ c. almond milk
1 c. raspberries, fresh
¼ c. chocolate chips, organic, unsweetened

Directions:
Combine all ingredients in a blender and process until smooth.

Dessert in a Glass

½ c. almond milk
1 sm. banana
2 tbl. hazelnut butter or almond butter

1 tsp. cocoa powder
1 tbl. maple syrup

Directions:
Combine all ingredients in a blender and process until smooth.

Dreamy Mango Smoothie

¼ c. mango cubes
¼ c. orange juice

¼ c. avocado
1 tsp. freshly squeezed lime juice

Directions:
A day ahead of time puree one mango and freeze in ice cube trays. Combine all ingredients in a blender and process until smooth.

My Morning Smoothie

1 handful of spinach, 30 or so leaves
1 collard green leaf, ½ if it is large
1 kale leaf, 5 - 6 baby kale leaves
⅛ c. or less flax seed
⅓ c. blueberries, frozen
⅓ c. strawberries or mixed berries, frozen
1 apple, sliced
1 banana, broke in half
apple juice with no sugar or water

Directions:
Combine all ingredients in a blender, add apple juice or water to 1 ½ inch above ingredients and blend for 2 to 3 minutes to your desired consistency. Sometimes I add nuts or turmeric, or carrots if I have some in the freezer or left over in the fridge. This makes about 2 quarts, I drink it down till it's gone.

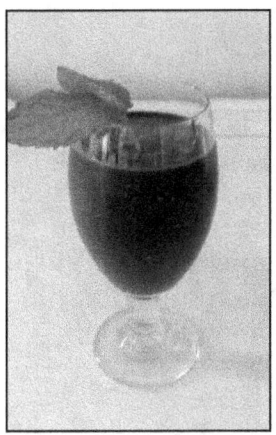

My Morning Smoothie

Strawberry-Peach Smoothie

2 c. strawberries, fresh or frozen
2 c. peaches or nectarines, coarsely chopped
2 oranges, coarsely chopped
1 c. kale. coarsely chopped, firmly packed
2 tbl. protein powder supplement with no sugar (optional, for an extra punch)

Directions:
Combine all of the ingredients in a blender and blend until smooth, 2 to 3 minutes, depending on your blender and how smooth you would like it.

South American Quinoa Drink

½ c. uncooked quinoa
2 apples, peeled, cored, quartered
1 tbl. vanilla

2 tbl. honey
½ tsp. cinnamon

Directions:
Cook quinoa in 2 c. water, bring to boil, reduce heat to low, cover & simmer 15 min. or until quinoa is tender, drain well. Return to pan and add almond milk, apples, honey and cinnamon, bring to simmer over med-high heat, reduce heat & simmer 5 minutes.
Take off heat, then add vanilla and blend in a blender until smooth. Serve hot, or re heat in the morning. Yum! I had something similar to this in the Philippines and LOVED it!

Watermelon Breeze

3 c. cubed watermelon   1 c. coconut water
squeeze of lime   sprig of mint

Directions:
Blend all ingredients in blender until smooth. So refreshing, and so
easy, makes 2 servings.

Frozen Smoothie Bags

Freeze the smoothie ingredients in a freezer zip lock bag. It takes
less than 30 minutes to put together enough bags for two weeks.
Having them ready in the freezer is so quick for rushed mornings.
Just empty a bag in a blender, add a liquid and blend!

Notes

_____

_____

_____

_____

_____

_____

_____

_____

_____

_____

_____

_____

_____

_____

_____

_____

_____

_____

_____

_____

_____

_____

Seasonings, Herbs, Spices

Jamaican Jerk Seasoning	122
Fajita Seasoning	122
Greek Seasoning	123
Italian Seasoning	123
Pumpkin Pie Spice	123
Ranch Dressing Mix	124
Seasoned Salt	124
Steak Rub	125
Taco Seasoning	125

Although there are a myriad of spice recipes out there, these are the ones I use. They are easy to put together and you know what is in them. I've adjusted them to my family's liking. We like more cinnamon and heat when it comes to our spices. You can adjust them to your taste.

Jamaican Jerk Seasoning

¼ c. onion powder
2 tbl. sea salt
2 tbl. thyme
2 tsp. ground allspice
1 tbl. cinnamon
1 tsp. cayenne powder (optional)

Directions:
Mix all items together and store in an air tight container.

Fajita Seasoning

¼ c. chili powder
2 tbl. sea salt, paprika
1 tbl. onion powder, garlic powder, cumin powder
1 tsp. cayenne pepper

Directions:
Mix all items together and store in an air tight container

Greek Seasoning

2 tsp. salt
2 tsp. dried oregano
1 ½ tsp. onion powder
2 tsp. garlic powder
1 tsp. cornstarch
1 tsp. pepper
1 tsp. dried parsley flakes
½ tsp. ground cinnamon
½ tsp. grated nutmeg

Directions:
Mix all items together and store in an air tight container. Use on meat or vegetables.

Italian Seasoning

½ c. basil, marjoram, oregano
2 tbl. garlic powder
¼ c. rosemary, thyme

Directions:
Mix all items together and store in an air tight container.

Pumpkin Pie Spice

¼ c. ground cinnamon
1 tsp. ground cloves
1 tbl. ground ginger, nutmeg, allspice

Directions:
Mix all items together and store in an air tight container.

Ranch Dressing Mix

¼ c. parsley
½ tsp. basil, pepper
1 tbl. dill, garlic powder, onion powder

Directions:
Mix all items together and store in an air tight container. Mix 1 tbl. with ⅓ c. greek yogurt and ¼ cup coconut milk.

Seasoned Salt

¼ c. onion powder, garlic powder, black pepper
2 tbl. chili powder, dried parsley
3 tbl. paprika
1 tbl. red pepper, ground
½ c. sea salt

Directions:
Mix all items together and store in an air tight container.

Steak Rub

¾ c. chili powder
2 tsp. dry mustard
¼ c. paprika
2 tsp. ground coriander
¼ c. cumin
2 tsp. pepper
2 tsp. salt
1 tsp. cayenne pepper

Directions:
Mix all items together and store in an air tight container. This will be warm, you can add 1 tbl. honey just before you rub it in for a sweeter taste.

Taco Seasoning

¼ c. chili powder, cumin powder
1 tsp. oregano powder, pepper
1 tbl. garlic powder, onion powder
2 tsp. sea salt

Directions:
Mix all items together and store in an air tight container. Use 3 tbl. with chicken, ground beef or turkey and cook as usual.

Herbs & Spices

Chicken
- *Dried herbs and spices:* thyme, rosemary, coriander, marjoram, sage, oregano
- *Fresh herbs:* thyme, rosemary, parsley, tarragon, marjoram, sage
- *Other:* lemon, garlic, soy sauce, ginger

Fish
- *Dried herbs and spices:* coriander, chili flakes
- *Fresh herbs:* chervil, tarragon, chives, dill, marjoram, cilantro
- *Other:* lemon, mustard, ginger

Pork
- *Dried herbs and spices:* sage, rosemary, thyme, marjoram
- *Fresh herbs:* sage, rosemary, thyme. oregano
- *Other:* mustard, garlic

Beef
- *Dried herbs and spices:* rosemary, thyme, basil
- *Fresh herbs:* rosemary, thyme, coriander
- *Other:* garlic

Lamb
- *Dried herbs and spices:*
- *Fresh herbs:* rosemary, thyme, parsley, mint
- *Other:* garlic

Steamed or Roasted Vegetables
- *Dried herbs and spices:* thyme, rosemary, oregano, marjoram, chili flakes
- *Fresh herbs:* dill, thyme, rosemary, oregano, marjoram
- *Other:* lemon, extra-virgin olive oil, butter

Potatoes
- *Dried herbs and spices:* rosemary, thyme
- *Fresh herbs:* rosemary, thyme, parsley
- Other: good extra-virgin olive oil, butter, pesto

Glossary

Almond Flour/Meal - Is made from ground sweet almonds. Almond flour is usually made with blanched almonds (no skin), whereas almond meal can be made both with whole or blanched almonds. The consistency is more like corn meal than wheat flour.

Amaranth Flour -Molecular biologists in Mexico studied the bioactive peptides in amaranth and, in 2008, were the first to report presence of a lunasin-like peptide in the protein in amaranth. Lunasin is a peptide previously identified in soybeans and is widely thought to have cancer-preventive benefits as well as possibly blocking inflammation that accompanies several chronic health conditions such as diabetes, heart disease, certain cancers, digestive-tract conditions and stroke. Amaranth offers a bonanza of near-complete protein and is much richer in iron, magnesium, and calcium than most grains.

Chickpea/Garbanzo Bean – is a legume. Hummus is the Arabic word for chickpeas. They are a nutrient-dense food, providing rich content of protein, dietary fiber, foliate, and certain dietary minerals like iron and phosphorus. Thiamin, vitamin B6, magnesium and zinc contents are moderate. Chickpeas have a Protein Digestibility Corrected Amino Acid Score of about 76 percent, which is higher than fruits, vegetables, and many other legumes.

Cocoa – Cocoa solids are a mixture of many substances remaining after cocoa butter is extracted from cacao beans. When sold as an end product, it may also be called cocoa powder, cocoa, and cacao.

Date Syrup – Syrup extracted from dates. Date Syrup is rich in monosacchirides glucose and fructose, so most of the sugar content is absorbed through the mouth which raises blood glucose levels quickly and immediately than other syrups. It is therefore highly suitable for people with hypoglycaemia or those with sucrose intolerance and those with pancreatic problems who have difficulty in absorbing disacchirides (a class of sugar)

Flax seed – is a food and fiber crop that is grown in cooler regions of the world. Flax seeds contain high levels of dietary fiber as well as lignin's, and abundance of micronutrients and omega-3 fatty acids. Studies have shown that flax seeds may lower cholesterol levels. And that flax seeds taken in the diet may benefit individuals with certain types of breast and prostate cancers.

Honey – A great natural source of carbohydrates which provide strength and energy to our bodies is known for its effectiveness in instantly boosting performance, endurance and reducing muscle fatigue of athletes during exercise. The glucose in honey is absorbed by the body quickly and gives an immediate energy boost, while the fructose is absorbed more slowly providing sustained energy. Honey has also been found to keep levels of blood sugar fairly constant compared to other types of sugar.

Mustard – made from the seeds of a mustard plant (white or yellow mustard, Sinapis hirta; brown or Indian mustard, Brassica juncea; or black mustard, B. nigra). The whole, ground, cracked, or bruised mustard seeds are mixed with water, salt, lemon juice, or other liquids, and sometimes other flavorings and spices, to create a past or sauce. The tastes range from sweet to spicy. The recipes are only for spicy, with NO SUGAR.

Dijon Mustard – originated in 1856, when Jean Naigeon of Dijon, France substituted verjuice, the acidic "green" juice of unripe grapes, for vinegar in the traditional mustard recipe. Most mustard from Dijon today contains white wine rather than verjuice. "Dijon mustard" is not a protected food name. While mustard factories still operate in Dijon and adjoining towns, most mustard described as "Dijon" is manufactured elsewhere. Even that produced in France is made almost exclusively from Canadian mustard seed.

Peppers, Chipotle – are smoked, dried jalapeno peppers.

Quinoa – Quinoa is a grain crop that is grown for its edible seeds. It is pronounced KEEN-wah. It technically is a pseudo-cereal, basically a "seed" which is prepared and eaten similarly to a grain. Quinoa was an important crop for the Inca Empire. They referred to it as the "mother of all grains" and believed it to be sacred. It has been consumed for thousands of years in South America. There are three main types of quinoa… white, red and black.

Stevia– is a sweetener and sugar substitute extracted from the leaves of the plant species Stevia rebaudiana. The active compounds of stevia are steviol glycosides, which have up to 150 times the sweetness of sugar, are heat-stable, pH-stable, and not fermentable. These steviosides have a negligible effect on blood glucose, which makes stevia attractive to people on carbohydrate-controlled diets. Stevia's taste has a slower onset and longer duration than that of sugar and some of its extracts may have a bitter or licorice-like aftertaste at high concentrations.

Turbinado Sugar – Also known as Real natural brown sugar, is a partially-refined sugar cane extract that's a healthier alternative to white and brown refined table sugars. Brown sugar is refined white table sugar with molasses added to it, it's not any better for you. I use "Now Real Food" Certified Organic Turbinado Sugar. It can be used as a 1 to 1 replacement for white sugar.

Xylitol – Xylitol is a naturally occurring carbohydrate, that looks and tastes just like regular table sugar. It is a natural sweetener that can be extracted from any woody fibrous plant material. Commercially it is extracted from renewable resources such as corn cobs, and also from less environmentally sustainable sources such as hardwood. Xylitol also occurs naturally in our bodies – in fact, an average size adult manufactures up to 15 grams of xylitol daily during normal metabolism. Pure xylitol is a white crystalline substance that looks and tastes like sugar.

Notes

_____

_____

_____

_____

_____

_____

_____

_____

_____

_____

_____

_____

_____

_____

_____

_____

_____

_____

_____

_____

_____

Notes

Recommended Readings

Heineman's Encyclopedia of Healing Juices, by John Heineman

Foundations for Healing, by Richard L. Becker, D.O.

The Fungus Link: Volume 1, by Doug A. Kaufmann

***Apple Cider Vinegar, Miracle Health* System**, By Bragg

Recommended Websites

www.bragg.com

www.greensmoothiegirl.com

www.nerdfitness.com

www.newportnaturalhealth.com

www.rawfoodlife.com

www.wikipedia.com

Buon Cibo

(Italian: Good Food)

www.ingramcontent.com/pod-product-compliance
Lightning Source LLC
Chambersburg PA
CBHW072248310526
45795CB00011B/393